THE WONDER PROTEIN DIET

Miracle Way to Better Health and Longer Life

THE WONDER PROTEIN DIET
Miracle Way to Better Health and Longer Life

Sidney Petrie
in association with
Robert B. Stone

Parker Publishing Company, Inc.
West Nyack, New York

Library of Congress Cataloging in Publication Data

Petrie, Sidney.
  The wonder protein diet.

  Includes index.
  1. High-protein diet. 2. Longevity--Nutritional aspects. 3. Nutrition. 4. Health. 5. Reducing diet. I. Stone, Robert B., joint author. II. Title.
RM237.65.P47   613.2'8   78-12691
ISBN 0-13-962498-8

Previous Books:

Fat Destroyer Foods: The Magic Metabolizer Diet

How to Reduce and Control Your Weight Through Self-Hypnotism

Hypno-Cybernetics: Helping Yourself to a Rich New Life

The Lazy Lady's Easy Diet: A Fast-Action Plan to Lose Weight Quickly for Sustained Slenderness & Youthful Attractiveness

Martinis and Whipped Cream: The New Carbo-Cal Way to Lose Weight and Stay Slim

Miracle Diet for Fast Weight Loss

Petrie's New Miracle-3 Guaranteed Diet

With Love to
David, Jacqueline, Danielle, Jackie and Stacey

Foreword

A healthy mind and a healthy body are the absolute requirements for both longevity and an ongoing enjoyable and productive life.

Poor nutrition, aided and abetted by stress, has been proven beyond doubt to walk hand in hand with chronic disease and early death.

Sideny Petrie has skillfully balanced the essential nutritional ingredients of foods and liquids with those of mental and emotional stability and produced a safe, medically sound, and important work in the arena of dietary health.

By following his techniques, the reader can fully savor the vitality and virility of everyday existence.

Robert Weintraub, M.D.

How This Book Can Add Years
to Your Life and Life to Your Years

"Eureka!" Archimedes exclaimed when he discovered the prinicple of floating objects which made him famous. I feel like shouting "Eureka!" too.

My discovery came quite accidentally, too, but I doubt if it will make me famous. However, it is of vital importance to every person alive today.

I am a nutrition consultant and behavioral therapist with a clinical practice consisting of clients referred to me by their physicians and from many other sources. Some have heart problems, others have high blood pressure or diabetes, or some other health problem that responds to improved eating habits. Many are simply overweight. Others are simply under-nourished.

In the process of helping these people as a para-medic, I have supplied them with easy, enjoyable ways to improve their health through simple changes in the way they eat and live.

Now, that all started about a quarter century ago. Today many of my clients look and feel younger than they did when they first came for assistance. Some, who came a decade or two ago, have more energy, more joie de vivre, more youthfulness in their body movements than when I first saw them.

At first my reaction was, "How well Mrs. T. looks" or "Mr. H. is really enjoying life."

Then I began to wonder. Did their brief visits to my office have something to do with Mrs. T.'s looking twenty years younger than her years, or Mr. H.'s youth-like vigor?

There were others who did not show this kind of improvement. I saw these people, too, because a number of them came back to my office five years later with the same problem or another kind of health problem.

I decided to ask some questions. That's when I made my discovery.

People like Mrs. T. and Mr. H. had adopted the healthful nutrition and healthful living information I gave them. The other returnees had not.

The program I was "prescribing" as a temporary measure to counteract a physical problem, when adopted permanently, was providing long-term results of inestimable value in terms of looks, aliveness . . . and longevity.

It is an easy and attractive program. My natural protein longevity diet calls for such actions as eating roast beef, drinking fruit juice, and taking a Sunday stroll.

It is based on the simple fact that the body needs certain foods. This "need" makes these foods taste good to us, naturally. We have, unfortunately, been taught to like some very poor foods. Unnatural food technology has been employed to "fool" our taste buds. We, therefore, need to get reacquainted with wholesome natural taste in good foods.

These foods are still good in taste. Yet, they are even better than good in taste. They do better than taste good because every cell in our bodies opens its mouth like a little bird for this naturally good food. As a result:

- Your body responds in higher and higher levels of resistance to disease.
- Your energy is boundless.
- You look years younger.
- You live longer.

Whenever somebody returns from a far away land and reports that he has seen centenarians living active, loving and working lives, I read the accounts avidly and see confirmation for my program. It is not new. It is just largely untried in 20th century United States.

It is an easy program. It involves delicious food, invigorating beverages, and new horizons in the "good life." It is all spelled out in the pages ahead—even my own special longevity drink. There is a glass of it in my hand now. I toast your youth, health, and longevity!

Sidney Petrie

ACKNOWLEDGMENTS

This book is based in part on research done by people throughout the world in various fields of nutrition, and sincere acknowledgement is made to those many dedicated men and women and their scientific and medical studies.

A great depth of appreciation is owed to Gertrude Loris, Charles Kazan and my wife Janet Petrie, for their assistance in research and manuscript preparation.

Contents

Chapter 1

You Can Live Longer

Eat as though your life depends on it.

It does!

You do not have to suffer from the typical ills of old age. Nor do you have to obey the "statistics" and quit this world at the end of your "life expectancy."

There is a correct way to eat that is even more enjoyable than the wrong way. This healthier diet not only increases your chances of a long life, but you begin to feel better right away.

You have more energy. Pains and aches disappear. You feel younger. You get more out of life, as you enjoy more years of life.

You know, of course, that some delicious dishes in our civilization produce unwanted penalties in poor health and even shortened lives. But there are ways to avoid civilized dietary "booby traps." There are ways you can enjoy your daily meals and snacks without any unwanted penalty. There are foods available that pack such a nutritional wallop they are likely to push you well past your present life expectancy.

Science is investigating several paths toward increased length of life for men and women. Researchers are experimenting with the lowering of body temperature, the revitalizing of the immunity systems of the elderly, and the transplanting of vital organs—all to help us live longer, perhaps to live indefinitely.

But what holds the greatest promise of longer lives for you and me are the dietary breakthroughs: ways to eat so you will live more years and healthier years. I am bursting with enthusiasm to tell you about these ways because I have seen them work miracles in my life and in the lives of countless others.

How many people would you guess there are now in the United States who are over 100 years of age. One thousand? Guess again—there are closer to 14,000! Medical science has extended our life expectancy. Still, for a time, medical science "forgot" and is now beginning to recall, an important adjunct to the medicine: food.

In food, nature provides man with all he needs to live a long and healthy life. There are foods that soothe upset stomachs, foods that lower blood pressure, foods that quiet nerves, foods that increase resistance to disease, and foods that make you sleep better.

I call them "wonder" foods.

On the pages ahead you will find menus and recipes using these "wonder" foods. They are delicious foods in their natural, savory flavors—every bit as "gourmet" as less healthy foods.

Yet they do more than just taste good. They make your body feel good.

"Wonder" foods go to work on any ailment or misery by providing the body with what it needs to correct the cause of the trouble. As a result, when you enjoy "wonder" foods, you enjoy better health.

You relieve aches and pains. You prevent illnesses. You live long.

Lest you confuse medical science with food technology, let me state here and now that when I use the word "food," I am not referring to items like the new synthetic seafood or synthetic pecans. I don't mean the egg substitute that is now turning up in restaurant salads throughout the country—consumers are unaware that it comes from a test tube, not a chicken!

Some health care specialists may care little what you eat, much less whether it is imitation food or real food, but those who are aware of the importance of nutrition are sticking to eggs from chickens, fish from the sea, and pecans from trees.

Nutrition-conscious professionals appreciate nature's products. They see the different effects of living foods and dead foods on health and longevity.

They see the health difference between vitamin and mineral-rich foods and refined or depleted foods.

And they see the health difference between people who follow natural protein-rich life styles and people who follow disease-ridden, fat-rich and starch-rich life styles.

Yes, I am talking about such nutritional foods as spinach, that we were all told was good for us. Yes, I am talking about the apple we have grown to respect. But I am also talking about scores of other delicious foods that we tend to walk by in the supermarket because they do not receive the flamboyant displays that less healthy foods receive. Leading the parade of longevity foods are the natural low-fat proteins, like fish, chicken, veal, lamb, and beef. Following close behind are whole grains, fresh fruits and fresh vegetables. But there are many more foods packed with life-giving power. I'll tell you about these.

HOW TO LIVE LONGER BY SWITCHING KEY FOODS

In parts of Scandinavia, where margarine is used instead of butter, the life expectancy of people is several years longer than in European countries to the south where butter is favored over margarine.

In the past twelve years 8,000 men of Japanese descent in Hawaii have been monitored along with 2,000 men of Japanese descent in California and 2,000 in Japan. The rate of coronary heart disease of the men in Hawaii was twice that of the men in Japan, and the men in California were dying off even faster.

The main reason? Animal fat. Yes, there were other variables, like physical activity and cigarette smoking, but, as reported, the men in Hawaii ate animal fat in greater amounts than in Japan and the men in California ate it in even greater amounts, leading to greater cholesterol content in the blood, high blood pressure and obesity—all killers.

We will be addressing ourselves to fat on the pages ahead, animal fat in particular. We will be exchanging one kind of fat for another kind of fat and winding up with a profit: years of life.

At the Longevity Institute in Santa Barbara, California, a developmental engineer named Nathan Pritikin, himself once a heart patient, has developed a program that is helping people to halt their angina and chest pains and return to work. Men with coronary problems are being treated at a private sanitarium and leaving in a couple of weeks able to resume normal activities free of pain. The key aspect of the treatment here is diet, and the key change in the diet is dropping the fat content from the ordinary 40 percent that is common to American eating ways down to ten percent. Sugars and salt are also dropped.

When we address ourselves to "killer fat," we will be switching not only from one kind of fat to a less dangerous kind, but we will be switching from fatty foods to non-fatty foods.

Living longer does not have to mean eating less, just eating differently, switching from one kind of food to another. I promise you a taste profit to boot.

Martin L., 46, made these switches away from fat. An accountant, he was eating fat-rich foods and becoming health-poor. He was not engaging in the kind of physical activities that his diet was supporting, so the excess was winding up on his girth and inside his arteries. He was mentally and physically "logey." He felt older than his years.

Martin switched from butter to margarine and from beef and pork to veal and chicken breasts. He did not give up gourmet lunches with his clients or his two martini dinners. Within two weeks, he reported to me he had more spring in his step and more mental alertness. He also had lost five pounds.

Animal fat produces cholesterol. Cholesterol can line the circulation system, increasing the work load on the heart. It closes some smaller veins and arteries altogether, causing poor circulation to parts of the body and, when the brain is involved—results in signs of senility.

There are several other switches away from one type of food "killer" to another type of food that add instead of detract from your years. The thrust of eating right is a process of selecting from a large variety of "wonder" foods.

"WONDER" FOODS FOR LONGER LIFE

Did you know that sardines are exceptionally high in nucleic acids, now considered by many experts to be of longevity-promoting value?

Did you know that yogurt is a natural antibiotic and considered to be the main nutritional secret of the long-lived Soviet Abkhasians?

Did you know that sourdough bread has none of the shortening (fat) in other breads that really shortens life but instead has lactic acid, a longevity promoting factor not found in other breads?

People who are aware of these and other health-promoting foods are living with more energy, more productivity, and more years.

I will share with you the secrets of longevity of many areas of the world where centenarians are not tourist attractions but normal productive members of their society.

I will list the "wonder" foods that are uniquely responsible for the health and vigor in these areas, and will demonstrate how you can include these foods in your menus and recipes.

I will give you the information you need to plan your own "wonder" casseroles, drinks, and dishes that pour vitality into your body.

We will be neither immortalists nor "inevitabilists." An immortalist is one who believes life can continue indefinitely whatever he does. An "inevitabilist"—a word invented by Malisoff—is one who is not willing to do anything to prevent death's advent.

I believe we can add many years to our lives or subtract many years from our lives by what we eat and drink. That puts me somewhere in-between an optimistic "inevitabilist" and a pessimistic immortalist.

What we eat and drink used to be a part of medical practice. The family physician would say, "get off sweets and starches" when he wants you to lose weight. Today, people try other ways of losing weight. There are pills for getting rid of water from the body and for depressing the appetite. There is even surgery to cut off unwanted pounds and shorten the digestive tract to prevent full digestion of the glutton's intake.

Heart patients once had to cut fat intake and lose weight. Today fat reduction seems to be considered less important by many heart specialists than the administering of a protocol of medicines to control the pain and other symptoms.

Instead of advising about food, too many doctors are, in effect, saying, "Eat what you think is right for your health and pleasure. If something goes wrong, we'll find a medical way for you to live with it or a surgical way for you to live without it."

So we are on our own. You and I must eat right in order to live longer. We must discover which are the "killer" foods. And we must get to know the "wonder" foods.

PROTEIN—"WONDER" FOOD NO. 1

Mary E., a school principal in her late thirties, was missing several days of work practically every month. She had colds, back aches and headaches,—nothing that her doctor could alleviate except through aspirin or other pain relievers. She was also overweight with 203 pounds on her five feet eight inch frame. Her doctor suggested she lose weight. That is when she came to my office. "My absences are interfering with teacher morale. I'll even go on a diet and lose weight if I have to."

I asked Mary to kaleidoscope for me a few days of her meals. It was a picture of coffee and "danish" breakfasts, school lunches, and "TV" dinners. It was obvious that even though she was overweight, she was undernourished. If she kept up her eating habits for another ten years, Mary would in important ways be starving to death. She would have some real problems for the doctor to treat.

Mary's body was being protein starved. It was also receiving more carbohydrates than a construction worker needed but fewer vitamins and minerals in those carbohydrates than her body required.

Mary did not have to go on a diet. All she had to do was switch foods. She switched from "danish" in the morning to bacon and eggs. She brought fresh fruit and gave up the school lunch canned variety. She switched to large portions of fresh fish, crisp fresh salads, and more fresh fruit or gelatin desserts.

The big switch was to protein. Mary doubled up on her daily protein intake at the expense of fats and carbohydrates, especially empty carbohydrates.

At the end of one month, Mary had lost 11 pounds. She continued to lose about five pounds a month for several months until she reached 165,—still somewhat overweight. But Mary's miseries completely disappeared. She had more energy. She was able to work on improving teacher and student attendance without guilt about absences of her own. Morale improved.

Another problem caused by poor diet is aging. Aging can start at 40 when bones not properly fed can lose substance. And bone deterioration, says Dr. Stanley M. Garn, professor of nutrition and anthropology, is the key to aging. The keys to proper feeding of your bones is adequate daily supplies of protein, minerals and vitamins.

Protein is from the Greek word meaning to "take first place." It is appropriately named. It is our number one food. Our entire body, except for the load of fat we may be storing, is made mostly of protein, from skin and muscles right through to the marrow of our bones. Protein-starved bodies sag, bulge, creak and ache. Protein-nourished bodies are firm and erect.

Hair, nails and internal organs all need protein to keep in repair. Brittle hair and break-prone nails are in need of natural protein. You cannot see the lack-luster look of internal organs, but you can feel their lack-luster performance. Protein nourished hair and nails take on a new resiliency; internal organs take on new harmonious functioning.

We can survive on minimum amounts of fats and carbohydrates. But we cannot survive without our full protein requirements.

Your body cannot make protein out of other kinds of food. It cannot transform fats or carbohydrates *into* protein.

However, your body *can* make fats and carbohydrates *out of* protein. Assuming the presence of adequate minerals and vitamins, a body can "manufacture" the fats and carbohydrates it needs to survive, but it cannot "manufacture" one ounce of protein—its priority food.

Where then do we get protein? Nature has given us a variety of sources. There are animal proteins and plant proteins. On the pages ahead, you will learn the best sources of proteins for the human body and how to incorporate them in your culinary life style for longevity.

THE COMMON DENOMINATOR OF CENTENARIANS

Tinei Sua Paia, born in Western Samoa, died in 1977 at the age of 105. He was survived by 119 descendants, including 53 grandchildren, 49 great-grandchildren and three great-great-grandchildren. He was a high priest in the Church of Jesus Christ of the Latter-day Saints (Mormon). As such, he did not smoke or partake of alcoholic beverages, nor did he drink stimulants such as coffee or tea.

True or false?—People who do not smoke or drink coffe, tea, or alcoholic beverages always live longer than people who drink such beverages? Answer: False.

Many centenarians have drunk moderate amounts of coffee or tea all their lives, and there is now medical evidence showing that moderate amounts of alcoholic beverages contribute to health.

Lebai Omar, a teacher of "Silat," the Malaysian art of self-defense, is 117 years old. He was married 17 times and divorced as many times.

True or false?—All people who have an active sex life with many partners live longer. Answer: False.

Many centenarians have lived with only one spouse during their life time and many have even been inactive sexually for a portion of their later life. Sexual activity and longevity do not appear to be related.

George Lycurgus died several years ago at the age of 101. Born in Sparta, Greece, he came to the United States as a young man and worked in his brother's salmon cannery on the west coast. Later he bought and managed the Oyster Grotto in the San Francisco Bay area, frequented by the famous and the rich. Later he moved to Hawaii and ran and Sans Souci, noted for its excellent food.

True or false?—People who east oysters, lobsters, poultry, meat and seafood live longer. Answer: True.

One common denominator of people who outlive other people is: protein. It can be in the form of fish or poultry or lean meat or natural grains that are combined to give complete proteins (more about which grains these are and how to combine them on the pages ahead). Natural proteins are the key to longevity.

This is not to say that natural protein will immunize you from all serious diseases. It will not. But should you contract a serious disease, your protein-nourished body will be more resistant to it, and you will recover more rapidly. This is not to say that natural protein will prevent you from being in an accident or some other disaster, but even if this should befall you, natural protein can help you recover.

Nor is this to say that there are no other keys to longevity. Certainly live foods, brimming with vitamins and minerals are essential to life and longevity.

So is exercise and fresh air.

So is mental health.

But natural protein is in "first place."

OTHER "WONDER" FOODS
THAT ADD YEARS TO YOUR LIFE

In Toledo or Walla Walla, a centenarian could be a tourist attraction. There is a place, however, where the centenarian is commonplace. It is a place where cancer is unknown, where there is no rush, no stress and strain, and where wholesome food grows in unsprayed, unchemicalized, natural abundance.

That place is Hunza. It is a tiny area sandwiched between India, the Soviet Union, China and Afghanistan. It is bounded on all sides by snowy mountains wth high passes and rivers.

A 1973 survey sponsored by the National Geographic Society and led by Dr. Alexander Leaf established that Hunza is an octo-generians' paradise and a centenarians' utopia. Recently, a world-wide UNESCO-sponsored report confirmed that Hunza was free from cancer—it is believed to be the only such place on earth.

Hunza people work all their long years. Clad in their cotton or wool robes and trousers, they exude vitality, energy and health. They love to sing and dance, even at 100. They eat food rich in protein, minerals and vitamins. Their protein comes from poultry and lamb, their main sources of animal protein as well as from dairy products such as clabbered milk and from grains.

Their vitamins and minerals come from fresh fruits such as apples, apricots, pears and grapes and from a variety of leafy vegetables.

There are no condominiums or cottages for rent in Hunza. There are no airports. In fact, it can almost be said, "You cannot get there from here."

And so traveling to Hunza is not available as an escape from civilized stress and civilized synthetic food.

You must make a Hunza-land out of where you are. It may not be a place as free of dust and pollution. It may not be a place as quiet and tranquil.

But wherever you live, you can obtain the same "wonder" foods that keep the Hunza men and women going.

Take spinach. Intuitively our grandparents knew it was good for them. You had to eat your spinach, or else . . .

According to a recent analysis reported in Environmental Engineering News, spinach has at least 30 minerals and trace elements. Many of these are essential to vital organs but still not that easy to come by.

The public image of spinach as a source of iron does not do it justice. Yes, it is a good source of iron. But it is also a good source of:

Potassium	Zinc
Phosphorous	Uranium
Manganese	Cadmium
Copper	Cobalt
Chromium	Thallium
Calcium	Boron
Aluminum	Nickel
Strontium	Lanthanum
Thorium	Rubidium
Antimony	

As you read these mineral names, some of your cells are reaching out in anxious expectation. "Just what I need."

Take apples. Intuitively our grandparents taught us that "an apple a day keeps the doctor away." Today, that is just as true as it ever was with two possible modifications: (1) Since today doctors don't make house calls, you might switch that to "keeps us away from the doctor;" and (2) Since some apples are not the same as they used to be with spraying and breeding, less for nutrition than for taste and appearance for better marketability, switch that to "A certain kind of apple a day . . ."

Archeologists have discovered evidence that Stone Age inhabitants of Central Europe ate apples. In Biblical days, apples were being eaten and given favorable "publicity." "Johnny Appleseed," born John Chapman, might have been the first advocate of natural health. A traveling missionary, he walked throughout Ohio and Indiana in the 1800's preaching spiritual and physical health as he planted apple trees and passed out seeds as he preached the gospel.

Apples contain vitamin A and C as well as being a good source of calcium. But new varieties of apples have fewer of these nutrients than the kind old folks remember, like Winesaps and Roman Beauties. Today's Red Delicious might be redder and sweeter, but redness and sweetness are qualities that increase impulse buying not longevity.

According to Dr. L. L. Schneider, "Apples have a regulating effect on the entire digestive system."* He points to the apple's pectin, a complex colloidal substance, and its phosphorous as the chief apple components which aid digestion.

Apples and spinach are "wonder" foods. They are nature's gift to man. They can add years to your life, all else being equal.

I mention these two "wonder" foods in particular because they have had good "press." You cannot argue against spinach or apples. Through the ages, their nutritional value has had strong public acceptance and support.

Occasionally, some nutritionist likes to make headlines by knocking a popular concept. He may say, "I have seen no evidence that this, that, or the other food promotes health." But I have seen no evidence that they have dared say this about apples or spinach.

---

*"Old Fashioned Health Remedies that Work Best", Parker Publishing Co., Inc., West Nyack, N.Y.

On the other hand, there seems to be some "wonder" foods that nutritionists lie in wait for. If I were to mention apricots, for instance (and I hereby mention apricots loud and clear), a score of statements might quickly appear to the effect that, "I have seen no evidence that apricots promote health."

To this I would reply, "Take a trip to Hunza-land and look at the people there. They attribute their longevity to the apricot."

And were I to mention buttermilk—again I hereby mention buttermilk resoundingly—then, "I have seen no evidence . . ." statements would again be made.

This time I would have to send them on a trip to the Caucasus Mountains of Russia where the Abkhasians proclaim buttermilk their favorite and attribute to this lactic acid milk much of the credit for their astoundingly long lives.

Some doctors may deny the value of "wonder foods" in adding years to life, but these foods are supported by professionals who take non-medical approaches to health care. Nutritionists take the view that food is your best medicine.

They believe that eating the right food every day is better than taking the right medicine every day. They believe, too, that the right food every day can possibly prevent or reduce the need for medicine.

My experience with thousands of clients seeking to improve their health convinces me that the wrong foods can take years off your life, and the right foods can add years to your life.

In the chapters ahead, I will give you both sides of this picture. I will give you the negative side concerning food additives, food preservatives and foods deprived of their original natural nutritives. I will tell you the foods to avoid.

At the same time I will, of course, emphasize the delicious foods that add energy, zest and productive years to your life—not only "wonder" foods, but everyday foods that supply what the cells of your body open their little mouths for.

THE LOWLY HAMBURGER— A FIRST CLASS NATURAL PROTEIN FOOD

Americans eat about a million pounds of hamburger meat daily. It is one of the most convenient and inexpensive ways to add protein and other nutrients to your face.

It also tastes good.

Yes, chopped meat is on the Natural Protein Longevity Diet. It is just one of the many meats that you enjoy now which will continue on your menus. There may be some changes recommended—such as the fat content of the hamburger meat you buy, the way you cook it, and the way to order hamburgers when eating out.

Salivary juices start flowing just at the mention of chopped steak so, lest I cause you to stew in your juice, let me give you some tips on hamburger meat.

First, I don't care whether your steak is chopped or unchopped. Porterhouse steak or flank steak, chopped or not, are good sources of nucleic acids, believed to have longevity-promoting value.

Chopped or not, beef needs to be trimmed of fat. While the protein should be feeding your cells, the fat could be clogging the pipes that bring the protein to your cells.

Supermarkets often label their ground beef as ground round or ground chuck, etc. These can bring premium prices. But the extra cost is not due to extra value necessarily. It is like offering chicken parts: the breasts bring one price, the thighs another and both prices are higher than the price of whole chicken. That is because the seller is performing an extra service by providing you with the chicken you like best.

There is no more or less nutrition in one kind of ground steak than another, except—The exception is fat content. Buy the lowest fat content in ground meat regardless of from what cut of the animal it is taken.

There may be an advantage or two in grinding your own steak. You are in control. Added profit to the seller comes from more fat. Added profit to you—in longevity—comes from less fat. If you grind you own, you can trim the meat before putting it through your home grinder.

Grind only what you intend to use. In the refrigerator, ground meat loses moisture and gains bacteria. Freshly ground meat used immediately tastes better and is safer. Even in the freezer, meat deteriorates. Fat grows rancid. Meat that is intact resists bacterial invasion better than ground meat. Freshly ground meat is best, and it is most freshly ground when you are the grinder.

You can also use an old restaurant trick: as you grind the chunks, add a little ice water. This is against the law for supermarkets or butchers as it adds to the weight and opens up a way to cheat, but when you do it, it is not only legal, it adds to the taste by preventing too much drying out in the cooking process.

Electric meat grinders are often just another attachment for electric food processing appliances. Or they are a separate plug-in appliance. Clean carefully after each grinding.

Be fat-conscious when cooking hamburgers, too. Broiling is better than pan frying. Either way, be sure that the melting fat has a way to drip away from the meat.

Start thinking of ways to add new zest to the burgers. How about mixing in some chopped onions? Or adding an ounce of Marsala wine?

But, I'm getting ahead of our story.

YOU CAN BEGIN TO LIVE LONGER TODAY

The late Paul Bragg, founder of health food stores and consultant to movie stars way back in silent film days, was 95 when he died in 1976. He was still going strong right up until the end,— lecturing, traveling around the world, jogging, swimming, and dating women.

After one of his last lectures, he was leaving, still surrounded by members of the audience, each with a special question to ask. One elderly man held the door of the elevator so he could ask his question, "Is it too late for me to start?"

"It is never too late. Start today!" roared Bragg as the door closed.

You may be 8 or 80. It does not matter. The diet in this book will help you to conquer illness and to add health and years to your life.

Come with me along the path to longevity. Investigate with me the foods that harm and the foods that help. Discover with me youth potions and life elixirs. Correct with me the food preparation methods that are robbing your body of life-giving nutrients. Plan with me the menus to live by with new taste enjoyment over your extended years.

Enjoy your new, slimmer, more youthful look. Enjoy your new energy. Enjoy your new peace of mind.

Not tomorrow. Today. The first day of the rest of your longer life.

Chapter 2

How to Stop Aging and Start "Youthing"

In the Russian Black Sea port city of Odessa, an unusual experimental program has been in progress since 1960. A group of 25 people have been given periodic injections of a special serum and, according to Dr. Alekhper Mekhtiev, chief medical officer of the Azerbaijan region and one of Russia's leading experts on aging, the aging process has been completely halted.

In an interview with Henry Gris, senior roving editor of the *National Enquirer,* Dr. Mekhtiev, supported by Dr. Abram Mintz, deputy director of the Soviet Union's Central Gerontology Institute, told how the injection program has been conducted. The serum is prepared basically from the human placenta and fortified with certain additives.

In 1966 the Institute selected twleve healthy people aged 45 to 60: six men and six women and thirteen people aged 61 to 89: seven men and six women. The first group was selected because they were showing premature signs of aging. Now, 12 years later, these people look exactly as they did then. The signs of aging have not been reversed but they have been halted in their tracks, according to the two Soviet doctors.

The 25 people have enjoyed "extremely good" health. In

fact, health complaints ceased three years after the treatments began.

The Russians expect to expand the project soon to 200 participants and infer that, hopefully, the therapy can then be made available to people all over the world. Now, brief news items from the Middle East indicate the similar research is going on there.

Meanwhile, it is doubtful that the details of the serum will be released. All we know is that the placenta is dried and powdered and certain other ingredients added.

The placenta is the organ by which the human unborn infant is attached to the inside of the womb and through which the infant's bodily needs are supplied.

The volunteers are given daily injections for 45 days and then go 45 days without the injections.

The placenta is tissue charged with human survival. The unborn infant depends on it. Just as heart cells are "programmed" to be heart cells, placenta cells are "programmed" to foster the survival of the youthful embryo.

Wheat has its germ. Plants have their seeds and nuts. Vegetables have their sprouts. Fish have their roe (and their sardines). Food associated with life in its initial stages seems to have an extra charge of energy that life thrives on. The placenta seems to be the human counterpart.

We can live longer. All we need to do is find a way to feed the cells of the body with foods that maintain cell birth and cell vitality.

When cells lose their vitality and are not replaced with newborn cells, the aging process has begun.

THE ANATOMY OF AN OLD MAN (OR WOMAN)

Let us take an inside look at this aging process. We know only too well what growing older looks like from the outside. In order to understand how best to slow the aging process with proper nutrition, we need to go inside the human body, down to the cell level.

The latest research points to a growing malfunctioning as the years go by in each human cell, in the relationship between DNA and RNA.

DNA is Deoxyribonucleic Acid. RNA is Ribonucleic Acid.

DNA is the primary bearer of genetic information. This information enables the cell to live its life as a liver cell or a skin cell. When cells divide, the DNA must, in effect, divide too—repeat itself. This it does through the RNA.

This transfer from DNA to RNA begins to fail with the years. Cell renewal by division becomes faulty. The look and feel of old age begins.

The so-called elderly or aged presently make up 10 percent of the U. S. population. It is not a statistic computed by chronological age but rather by the aging process.

We all have a stake in getting the DNA and RNA to keep talking.

Maybe that stake should be spelled steak.

Nucleic acids in our diet help to keep our cells supplied with DNA and RNA. Natural proteins contain those nucleic acids in varying amounts.

We read news reports about people like Ervin S., a Californian who goes dancing twice weekly. He is 95. His dancing partners at the Friendship Club on Saturdays and Gay 90 S Club on Wednesdays say he is a good dancer and spry for his age. We also read how Maud T. renews her driver's license every February. She is 104 and is one of about a dozen licensed drivers in California who are over 100 years old.

Senior citizens continually make the news. To be able to dance, drive, think philosophically, and be interviewed intelligently, these oldsters have something going for them—their nucleic acids.

In 1974, the National Institute on Aging was created by an Act of Congress. Its work has largely centered on the medical and social problems that arise from aging rather than on an attack on aging itself.

Now, some three years later, the Institute is devoting some of its attention to the prevention of mental and physical deterioration. At a recent seminar sponsored by the Institute, Dr. Eleanor Schlenker, a nutritionist with the University of Vermont, told of an interesting finding.

In 1948, a study had been made in Michigan of a group of women. The study was picked up again in 1972. The subjects in that initial study who had died were found to have had lower intakes of protein and ascorbic acid (vitamin C) than survivors. Now, those survivors, re-studied, were found to have decreased their intakes of *total calories*, decreased their intake of *fat*, and decreased their intake of carbohydrates, while maintaing an adequate intake of proteins, vitamins, and minerals.

Attendees at the seminar where Dr. Schlenker made this report should have stood up and applauded. Copies of the report should have been widely circulated and publicized. Instead, these remarkable findings on aging were just politely received, and the meeting went on to the next speaker.

I carry the message to you on these pages. To be a "survivor," you must: lower your caloric intake, lower your fat intake (especially your intake of animal fat—more about this later), and lower your carbohydrate intake (expecially your intake of nutritionally "empty" carbohydrates—a lot more about this later, too). To replace the intake of these food elements, add more natural protein, vitamins, and minerals.

LONGEVITY STARTS IN THE KITCHEN

The greatest advance toward bodily immortality some people believe can be made in the kitchen.

Here are the goals that should be before every longevity-minded meal planner and preparer:

- To use the best natural proteins available.
- To provide the most nutritive fresh fruits and fresh vegetables available.
- To keep fat, especially animal fat, to a bare minimum.
- To favor "wonder" foods and beverages.
- To make vitamin and mineral supplements always available on the table.
- To cook the foods in a way that does the least damage to nutritive content.
- To include a variety of whole grains.

- To avoid prepared foods that contain chemicals, preservatives, colorants and other unnatural additives.
- To avoid white sugar and salt as much as possible.
- To provide a balanced diet.

You might call these "The Ten Commandments" for healthful eating.

They are not the whole story to longevity. But they constitute one giant step in that direction.

I am going to tell you how to put each one of these precepts into practice in your kitchen, for life-extending enjoyment of your daily meals.

You have my solemn promise that you will be sacrificing no "good taste." Everything you eat will, in effect, taste better to you. At the same time, you will not be "hypnotized" into buying the kinds of prepared sugar-sweetened foods that may save you minutes today but cost you days off your life later. You will be able to realize what "good food" means.

You also have my solemn promise that as your body begins to receive through this fare the advantages of natural protein, live foods, and the vitamins and minerals it needs, you will feel the difference. You will have more spring in your step, more *joie de vivre*, more gleam in your eyes.

EACH DAY YOU WAIT
MAY COST SEVERAL DAYS OF LIFE

In the October 10, 1975 issue of *Science*, evidence was presented from laboratory studies by M. H. Ross of the Fox Chase Cancer Clinic in Philadelphia and by G. Bras of the Rijks University in Utrecht, Netherlands, that overeating shortens life span, and the earlier in age th overeating the shorter the life. These studies were conducted on rats.

I hesitate to point to animals to make a conclusion about humans. But scientists are doing it everyday, and it seems to be valid more frequently than not.

We have known of the dangers of overeating all along. Insurance companies' actuarial tables have always equated overweight pounds with shorter life, and the longer the extra baggage was toted, the quicker the demise.

However, the Ross-Bras research contains an interesting sidelight. The main thrust was to show the relationship between total caloric intake and life span. This was confirmed. The 121 rats in the research project were allowed to select their own diet after their first 21 days of life. Then the amounts were monitored. The average life span of a rat is 630 days. These rats lived from 317 days to 1,026 days. The length was directly related to quantity of food, in fact quite dramatically.

But what also emerged was: those rats choosing a low protein diet early in life, were more likely to have short lives than the rats choosing a high protein diet. The rats that chose a high protein diet lived longer. This was especially true when the decision to eat lots of protein occurred before midlife. Later decisions were less productive.

"Diet is apparently the only way we know of to date," concluded Ross, "to increase the length of life of a warm-blooded animal."

PROPER DIET—THE LONG AND THE SHORT OF IT

We are talking in generalities. It is generally true that:

1. If you do not overeat and are therefore not overweight, you will live longer.
2. If you eat adequate natural protein, you will live longer.
3. If your daily intake includes vitamins and minerals, you will live longer.

It is also true, generally speaking, that the earlier in life you begin to observe these three general principles, the more years they will add to your life expectancy.

But there are also some specifics that you need to be aware of in order for these three truths to be true for you in particular.

Someone might be eating moderately, enjoying natural protein, vitamins and minerals in adequate amounts and yet succomb to a specific dietary inadequacy, possibly a deficiency in bran.

Now bran has no nutritive value. You cannot point to bran and claim it provides a single mineral or vitamin to the body. And it is not protein. It is nothing but roughage. However, therein lies its value.

Unfortunately, today bran has been removed from most of our wheat products. It is the outermost layer of the wheat kernel. It is not digestible. Yet it is one of the richest sources of roughage—natural food fiber which by its very indigestibility provides a valuable need to the human body. It cleanses the colon, causing shorter terms of contact between the tissue of the colon and the waste passing through it.

The body is a complicated organism. Man in all of his technology has not come close to producing a mechanism of such exquisite balance and such advanced processes.

Feeding this organism has not only the generalities we have pointed out, but also many specifics.

So as we proceed through the chapters ahead, we are going to be looking at both generalities and specifics. We are going to be taking both the bird's eye overview and the ant's eye view,—the long and the short of longevity.

SOME GIANTS IN THE FIELD
OF EATING RIGHT TO LIVE LONGER

Science is beginning to rediscover nutrition. This return to food awareness has been largely a process of the tail wagging the dog.

Thanks to the persistent work of a handful of proponents, the public has become conscious of the health protecting and health restoring potential of their daily fare.

It has been an uphill fight. The curative and restorative powers latent in food are nowhere near as strong, quick and dramatic as those in medicines and drugs. It may take weeks or months for acidophilus milk (explained later) to alleviate stomach distress, whereas an antacid over-the-counter preparation might do it in minutes.

But now people are realizing that empty calories might be quick and easy to put in their mouths and sweet to their taste, but these foods can produce long-term physical problems with a bitter after taste. Corrected by medicine, these unwanted after effects may seem to disappear dramatically, but what has really disappeared are the painful symptoms of a nutritional problem. Since the problem is still there, it will not take long for these symptoms or equal ones to re-appear. More medicine and drugs are taken, another respite occurs, and the cycle continues.

So the common sense of people has demanded an alternative. That alternative has been courageously delineated by such well known names as Adelle Davis whose eat right and cook it right books are lengend; Carlton Fredericks, whose voice on radio for decades, has made millions of people nutritionally aware; and Paul C. Bragg, whose concern led him to be one of the founders of America's physical fitness movement.

Perhaps the latter name, Bragg, has won the most acclaim because he put his teachings where his mouth was. He was a living example of his life extension precepts. Yes, he wrote about them, lectured on them, and taught classes in them. But his own body was a living testimony to these precepts.

All through his seventies, eighties, and nineties—ages that spell "finis" for most men—Bragg danced, jogged, loved, swam, and enjoyed life to the fullest.

If you were a visitor to Hawaii, his favorite place, during the 1960's or 1970's, you may have seen him on the beach at Waikiki surrounded by a hundred or more admirers, leading them daily through two hours of calisthenics, jogging, swimming, and a brief lecture on nutrition.

Bragg advocated raw fruits and raw vegatables. When he was not eating fish, poultry or meat, he was eating cheese, nuts, soy beans, and whole grains in order to supply his body with proteins.

He proclaimed the vital advantages of pure water, fresh air, sunshine, and natural "live" foods. He deplored the deadening of unnatural, devitalized foods and stimulating beverages.

His boisterous manner was controversial but it won him more friends than enemies. His real enemies were the purveyors of white flour and white sugar who he accused as America's public enemies number one.

"Don't panic—we're going organic," was his battle cry.

When Paul Bragg died of a heart attack in Florida in 1976, those who knew him intimately said this man of 95 had a body of 55 or 60.

Bragg reached millions in his lifetime. His contemporaries in the health food field reached more millions.

Now public pressure seems to be making some visible waves.

Alternatives to medical health care are being investigated, including the possibility of keeping well through preventive nutrition,—a longevity diet, if you will.

You can end pains and aches much more quickly than you imagine. They are ready to go away. They are like a baby crying. Feed the cells and organs of your body with natural protein and "wonder" foods and the "baby" stops crying.

WHY WOMEN LIVE LONGER THAN MEN

One key to longevity lies in the difference between the life expectancy of women as compared to men.

The insurance industry, our "bookies" in the game of life, have continuously made women the favorites in their "betting." The odds call for women living several years longer than men.

However, that difference shows signs of equalizing and the reason appears to be that women are leading lives more resembling those of men. In the battle for equality, women are losing their life expectancy advantage.

This points to factors that effect longevity which appear to be outside the realm of diet. Women eat the same food generally as do men whether at home or in the office. Now that they are in the office more and at home less, women are more subject to stress and anxiety. The factors that may have been causing the higher death rates of men in this century are now being shared by women.

One evidence of this is smoking. People under stress smoke more. Women are now smoking more than they did a decade ago before their battle for equality had been fully launched. Traditionally, more men have been smokers than women and this has accounted for an estimated 47% of the difference in life expectancies of men and women between the ages of 37 and 87, according to Dr. Charles Lewis and nurse Mary Ann Lewis, reporting in the *New England Journal of Medicine.* Now, more women are smoking and more women are dying of lung cancer.

Stress and anxiety brings about more than just the smoking habit. They yield the ulcer habit, the high blood pressure habit, and a multitude of health problems ranging from the psychosomatic to the functional, from the simple headache to the fatal heart attack.

It would be misleading of me to present my Protein Diet to you without also offering you guidance in handling some of the other factors that affect life expectancy. These factors are many. Some are inherited. Others are under our control. I cover the main factors under our control in the chapters ahead, with an entire chapter devoted to the most dangerous non-diet life shorteners: tension and anxiety.

Here women need to sit up and take notice as much as do men. Good nutrition makes us less vulnerable to life-eroding tensions and anxieties. But in Chapter X, I give you simple how-to instructions to insulate yourself effectively from stress,—how to remain in stressful situations without letting them "get to you."

CARDIOVASCULAR AGING—OUR CREEPING DEATH

Diet. Control of stress.

These are two contributions to your longer life that I make on the pages ahead—two that I have already mentioned. But there are more.

These two do not address themselves basically to one of America's most insidious killer: cardiovascular diseases. Yes, the reduction of animal fat is a great deterrent to cardiovascular troubles. And our diet handles that. But right now your tiny capillaries are getting blocked by poisons and residues in your food and drinking water.

It is like a creeping death.

These days it is starting earlier. Youngsters in their teens have been found to have blocked capillaries that interfere with brain functioning. This is getting to be a hostile environment, and it behooves me to see that while your body has stopped aging and started "youthing" by means of the Natural Protein Longevity Diet, some poisons don't creep into the picture and sabotage the plan.

Old age is a one-time experience. If we got a sample of old age in our youth in order to feel what it is like, we would take a lot better care of ourselves.

The lives of some old people are miserable. Take Charles H., aged 76, who suffers from painful arthritis, so much that he can hardly move. His wife Emily, is senile and has no control over urination or bowels.

Compare these people to a woman such as Khfaf Lasuria, 130, described by Alexander Leaf, M.D. in the January, 1973 issue of *National Geographic*. She was active around the house, able to sit on her porch and watch the world go by in the Soviet Union's Abkhasia. She was free of pain, in control of her body and her senses, and enjoying every day. Her physical activity kept her capillaries flushed.

Compare the wasting senility of Charles and Emily also with Markhti Tarkil, 104, of Duripshi, Abkhasia. He has taken a daily swim all his life, winter and summer in a chill stream down a steep trail a half mile from his home.

You can just see the surge of circulation this brings, his blood coursing through his capillaries and washing them clean for another day of life's enjoyment.

How about a gentleman named Tikhed Gunba? At 98 he still gathers tea leaves at the same volume he did decades ago. His father lived to be 125 and as Dr. Leaf put it, Tikhed Gunba has a lot of mileage left, thanks to the kind of diet and active life style he leads. He's kept his arteries soft and unclogged and his blood pressure at an enviable 104 over 72.

And so what you and I have embarked on is not only a diet of "wonder" foods to eat and other foods to avoid. It is also a program of fresh air, clean water, and healthful mental and physical activities.

THE TRUE BLESSING OF LONGEVITY

This program would be an exercise in futility if it did not have some exciting dividends which I can now divulge to you.

My clients report that every day is worth more to them than every before.

They report that their taste buds become more sensitive, and they are able to discriminate between foods that are just good and foods that are gourmet. They can enjoy food as never before. Other senses—of smell, sight, and touch—also improve.

They report that they can get more done in a day. Whether productivity means assembling, fixing, painting, or house work, they are able to soar through their tasks as if they took no energy. Gone are the tired feelings and the calendar or clock watching. Every day is a joy not an effort.

And I guess you're old enough for me to tell you, too, that my clients report heightened pleasure in their sex lives. Awakened senses and heightened gland activity seems to spell more fun in bed.

So the dividends of longevity are not experienced in fading years at the end of the line. They start when you start.

These dividends take you on a different path. It is not a path that leads to a hospital

Millions of Americans are in hospitals or are out-patients. Between 20 and 30 million require some kind of care in the mental health area. They suffer from alcohol and drug misuse, social isolation, physical handicaps, anger, depression and fear. Millions more will be out-patients or in the hospital tomorrow with physical problems that are festering today.

It is not so in other parts of the world. It is especially not so in those parts of the world where natural nutrition is a way of life.

Are you ready to discover what natural nutrition is?

No, it is not bland, tasteless and weird. It is not carrot sticks and lettuce leaves. It is not a routine, a discipline, or even a diet.

It is a way of selecting from a world of delicious foods in an intelligent way.

It costs nothing in enjoyment. It takes no will power because it powers itself once you give it a push.

In the next chapter, I will tell you how to provide that initial push.

Chapter 3

"Wonder Foods
for Your Longer Life

In this chapter we are going to get right down to the business of living longer.

This will be a capsuled course in natural nutrition for a healthier body and sharper mind.

Before going into the actual Natural Protein Diet in a later chapter, I now want you to understand the Diet's life-supporting ingredients.

When you finish this chapter you will, in fact, be able to create your own Longevity Diet. We will be discussing the three major components of food: protein, fat, and carbohydrate. We will discuss vital facts about each, such as the difference between a complete and incomplete protein; between saturated and poly-unsaturated fats; and between living versus "empty" carbohydrates.

We will also be introducing you to the "wonder" foods that are readily available but largely ignored, leading to a long, youthful, and healthy life on planet Earth.

THE PROTEIN: BASIC BODY ESSENTIAL

Our entire body is made mostly of protein from skin and muscles right through to the bones. Protein-starved bodies sag and bulge. Bodies well-nourished with protein are firm and erect.

The body cannot manufacture its own number one component. Protein cannot be synthesized from fats or carbohydrates. It cannot be created from the water we drink or the air we breathe.

Your body depends on you for its protein. Your decision concerning what to buy at the supermarket or what to order in a restaurant may seem about as important to you as what movie to go to or what TV channel to switch on. But, to the cells of your body, that food-buying decision is a matter of life and death.

Take your hair and nails. Brittle hair and nails are a sign of protein deficiency. Both take on new resiliency when protein in proper abundance is absorbed by your body.

Your vital organs suffer, too, from protein lack. They do not protest as quickly or as "loudly" maybe as hair and nails. Their protest is over a period of years and by the time you hear it, the damage may be irreversible.

A bottle of "Coke" may appear to give you a quick lift. But an order of calf's liver gives you a lift, too. It may not be as dramatic at the time, but the life provided by the liver eventually takes you right out of the life-limits of the actuarial tables into life-unlimiting longevity.

Protein foods build and replace hair, nails, skin, teeth, blood, heart tissue, lung tissue, kidney tissue, liver tissue, glands, brain, cartilage, tendons, muscle, hormones, enzymes, antibodies, and much more—all the way to the marrow of your bones.

Proteins are a mind-staggering complex of molecular forms that can be further sub-divided into twenty-two amino acids. While we can synthesize most of these amino acids in our own bodies, we need to obtain eight (valine, methionine, leucine, isoleucine, lysine, phenylanine, trytophane and threonine) from dietary sources.

A protein food is said to be complete if it contains these eight essential amino acids in the proper balance and proportion. Some good protein foods are not complete in themselves.

Beans have amino acids but not all. They are not protein as far as the body is concerned.

Corn has amino acids but not all because of incomplete unuseable protein.

Together corn and beans have all the amino acids. Together

corn and beans make a complete protein. The Mexicans have known this right along, at least intuitively.

Peanut butter is not a complete protein. Neither is bread. But together they supply what each lacks and form a complete protein. Kids must be intuitive, too.

Our main sources of complete protein are meat, fish, and poultry. Milk, cheese and eggs are also high in protein but another ingredient begins to enter the picture here: fat. In a moment, we will cover this category of food, but meanwhile we need to select *proteins that contain the least amount of fat.*

Fish gets a gold star. It is excellent protein with minimum fat. Poultry comes next, except duck and goose which are too fatty. Even chicken, guinea hen, and turkey have excess fat in the skin, and often, too, in the darker meat, like the thighs.

Finally, lean cuts of meat are excellent protein with lean beef and veal ranking high, especially the organ meats like liver, sweetbreads, kidney and brain.

On the bottom of the meat list as a source of protein is pork—too much fat.

Lamb is fine. So are the game meats like venison, when lean.

A friend of mine, Sam O., who loved to eat fat, suffered from mysterious bouts of indigestion which often led to bloating, considerable discomfort and sometimes nausea. Sam was not aided by the medication offered by his M.D. or by the various digestive drugstore potions. He was one of the very few customers of the Kosher deli who asked for a fat corned beef sandwich. Sam would also act as the human disposal for all leftover pieces of fat from the family meal, including his absolute favorite—chicken skin.

I insisted that Sam try for at least two weeks a low fat protein diet, consisting of fish, veal, poultry (without skin) and *lean* beef. The digestive upset disappeared after the first three days and brought him his first relief in years. The discomfort only returns when he forgets to restrict his fat intake.

There are so many cuts of lean meat available at the average meat counter that your menus are limitless. The Natural Protein Diet has practically unlimited choices available for exciting variety all through the years ahead. And years. . . and years.

THE CARBOHYDRATE: FRIEND OR FOE?

Carbohydrates are the energy foods. Our body needs energy in order to function. We need energy in order to have our bodies function.

The body can take in more carbohydrates than are immediately needed. Carbohydrates in excess are stored as fat. When energy is needed and no carbohydrates are being assimilated at the time, the body has two choices: it can convert its own protein into energy, or it can convert stored fat into energy.

Naturally, the body will first use its stored fat for energy before borrowing protein from its own tissues. So carbohydrates can be called protein sparing.

They also assist in the digestion and assimilation of other foods.

Carbohydrates are basically sugars and starches. They are in grains, fruits and vegetables. They are supplied by nature with extra nutritional bonuses: minerals and vitamins.

However, man has invented some ways to preserve these carbohydrate foods which deplete them of their nutritional bonuses. The results are pure carbohydrates devoid of any value except that of providing energy.

The more we eat of these "empty" carbohydrate foods—like white sugar and white flour—the less hungry we may appear to feel, but the hungrier our body is actually becoming.

We have temporary energy but we are a step closer to permanent rest.

The cells of our bodies must be fed if we are to remain healthy and alive.

An apple contains food for the cells of our bodies—lots of minerals and vitamins. But eat the apple out of a can called apple sauce and the "life" is out of your apple. It has been cooked out, chemicaled out, and sugared out. Net results—"empty" carbohydrates. If you count on such foods for your source of carbohydrates, you can count on "quick energy"—and a quick demise.

Raw apples. Raw fruits and berries. Raw vegetables or vegetables cooked in ways I will describe later that retain vitamins and minerals. These are the living sources of nutritive carbohydrates. Whole grains and brown rice are your friends.

Man profits from the white and depleted varieties only when he's in that business.

Like proteins, the family of carbohydrates have many components, but unlike proteins they are not incomplete of themselves. They do not need each other.

Here are the most common kinds of carbohydrates and their chief sources:

- Mono-, di-, and poly-saccharides (honey, fruits, and whole grains)
- Glucose (grape sugar)
- Galactose ("Yogurt" sugar)
- Fructose (fruit sugar)
- Mannose ("cherries")
- Sucrose (cane, maple sugar)
- Lactose (milk, sugar)
- Maltose (malt "grain" sugar)
- Starch (plant "sugar")
- Dextrins ("toasted bread" sugar)
- Glycogen (animal starch)
- "Indigestible Polysaccharides" (otherwise knowsn as fiber, bulk and cellulose)

FATTENING FATS—YOU CANNOT LIVE WITH THEM AND YOU CANNOT LIVE WITHOUT THEM

An Eskimo can live on a diet of blubber—some protein, lots of fat, no carbohydrate.

Most of us would not make it on such a diet. Fats are concentrated calories. One gram of fat provides nine calories of energy—more than twice as much as does one gram of carbohydrate or one gram of protein, each of which provides only four calories of energy.

Small amounts of fat are essential to the smooth functioning of the human body. Fat to us is like the oil that lubricates our car's engine and moving parts. Fat provides cushioning and insulation for vital organs. Fat aids in digestion and in the utilization of some other foods. And fat helps us to assimilate such vitamins as A, D, E, and K, which are themselves fatty substances.

The foods that provide our natural proteins, especially meat, poultry, fish, eggs, milk, and cheese contain enough fat to satisfy the needs of our bodies. The problem is that there may be more fat than we need. More fat than we need costs years off our lives.

An active life in the out-of-doors tends to burn up fat. But a diet high in fat in a lifestyle of heated rooms, and sedentary work, results in an oversupply. Fat deposits clog our arteries and line our vital organs with burdens of fat.

Excess fat—no matter where it deposits itself on our body—is anti-longevity.

Since excess carbohydrates become excess fat, these two foods in excess work against the realization of our full life longevity potential.

Richard B., 60, was in good health except for a few problems. He was thirty pounds overweight, looked older than his years, and had chronic digestive problems.

Then he began to get gallbladder attacks. The gallbladder concentrates the bile of the liver so it can digest fat better. Stones can form in the gallbladder. However, examination by x-ray could not confirm that Richard had stones.

In order to try to avoid acute gallbladder trouble, Richard gave up some of his favorite foods: heavy cream on his cereal and in his coffee, butter on his toast, eggs altogether (except the whites in cooking), and fatty meats.

He began to feel much better. Digestion improved. His weight began to drop. And his gallbladder gave him only minor "signals."

Then one day he was lunching at a steak house and saw on the menu that short ribs were the special of the day. A few minutes later, he was enjoying the tender meat and picking at the ribs.

The next morning at 2 a.m., Richard awoke with a gallbladder attack. By 7 a.m. he was hospitalized and being prepared for surgery.

The operation was a success in many ways. Richard no longer had a gallbladder to make stones that clogged tubes or to digest fat efficiently. So he really cut down on fat, with no more "detours" like the short ribs. Only a few years since the operation,

Richard looks ten years younger. His health is perfect, as reduced fat content in his body is yielding more efficient organ functioning.

The "high fat" way of eating has been an American way for too long. Nowhere in the rest of the world are people so beset with high fat problems as here. Now, however, the American people are beginning to change diets. People are eating leaner cuts of meat. They are switching to low-fat milk products. And they are turning away from lard, bacon fat, and butter and replacing them with margarine and vegetable oils.

This new awareness of danger in eating too much fat is related to knowledge of the danger of cholesterol. This is an ingredient in animal fats. Cutting down cholesterol means cutting down on fat.

This is a life-saving change. It can yield fewer gallbladder operations. It can reverse arterial clogging. And it can reduce premature death from heart disease.

Fats are made up of three different fatty acids: saturated, monounsaturated, and polyunsaturated.

If you consider fat as a chain of carbon atoms, then a fatty acid that has not more room for more carbon atoms is called saturated. This usually means it already contains more than 14 carbon atoms.

If a fatty acid can take on two more carbon atoms, it is called monounsaturated.

If a fatty acid can take on more than two carbon atoms, it is called polyunsaturated.

Nutritionally, all you need to know is that animal fats generally have a high proportion of saturated fatty acids which are less likely to be assimilated and more likely to be deposited where we don't want them. Color them cholesterol.

On the other hand, vegetable oils (oil is fat) are relatively low in saturated fats, low in cholesterol.

Ounce for ounce, saturated fats—like animal fat—are twice as likely to increase the cholesterol level in clogged arteries as nonsaturated fats are likely to lower it.

Monounsaturated fats, like peanut oil and olive oil, have no known effect on cholesterol levels.

The beneficial oils—the polyunsaturated oils that lower

cholesterol levels—are the vegetable and seed oils like soybean oil, corn oil, safflower oil, sunflower oil, and cotton seed oil.

Keep your eyes open for fat, especially animal fat. Cut your intake all you can.

Of course, none of our wonder foods are high in animal fat.

VITAMINS—THEIR MEANING FOR LONGEVITY

Vitamins are chemical compounds that stimulate healthful functioning of all the systems of the body.

Without vitamins, bones break, skin falls off, and organs fail.

Vitamins are non-fattening. A minimum daily supply of all the essential ones will put on a negligible 1/33 of an ounce. But they are worth a lot more than their weight in gold, in maintaining a high degree of good health.

New vitamins are constantly being discovered. At the present there are 23 known varieties from A (anti-infective) to Q (essential to blood clotting), B-1 (carbohydrate metabolism) to B-15 (anti-aging properties).

No one vitamin is more important than the other. All are needed together in the proper amounts and proportions that can best be obtained through that old standby: "A well-balanced diet."

Here are the essential vitamins currently identified:

> *Vitamin B-1 (thiamine)*—Required for proper carbohydrate metabolism, normal digestion and appetite. Also known as the "morale vitamin," thiamine helps smooth over everyday stresses and strains. It is the first of the so-called B-complex family.
>
> *Vitamin B-2 (riboflavin)*—Essential for the proper utilization of carbohydrates, fats and proteins. Promotes good vision and maintains healthy skin, hair and nails.
>
> *Vitamin B-6 (pyridoxine)*—Required for proper protein, fat and carbohydrate metabolism. Involved in antibody formation, the production of digestive juices and the maintenance of sound nerves.

Vitamin B-12—The "anti-anemia" vitamin, it helps build red blood cells. It also facilitates cell longevity and can therefore be considered an "anti-aging" vitamin.

Biotin—Possibly the most potent vitamin, a little goes a long, long way. Involved in the metabolism of proteins, fats and carbohydrates, it also facilitates cell growth and aids in the utilization of the B-complex in general. Deficiencies are rare.

Choline—Helps reduce serum cholesterol. Facilitates nerve transmission and is necessary for proper fat and cholesterol metabolism.

Inositol—In conjunction with choline, inositol helps reduce serum cholesterol and takes preventative action against hardening of the arteries. It is also involved with the metabolism of fats and cholesterol.

Folic Acid—Facilitates regular growth and reproduction of blood cells and generally shares the properties and duties of vitamin B-12.

Niacin—Required for the proper utilization and assimilation of proteins, fats and carbohydrates. Improves P.B.A. (Para-Aminobenzoic Acid) which is involved with protein metabolism, formation of red blood cells and more speculatively, restoring color to gray hair.

Vitamin A—Anti-infective, anti-allergic properties. Decreases serum cholesterol and helps detoxify poisons. Keeps skin smooth and soft, outside and inside (epithelial linings). Possibly helps keep precancerous cells from becoming cancerous.

Vitamin D—Anti-aging effects on the skin. Helps facilitate normal bone growth and maintenance.

Vitamin E—Acts as an antioxidant (prevents rancidity). Literally keeps your body from "spoiling." Current evidence suggests that vitamin E slows the aging process, helps prevent heart disease and (more speculatively) helps prevent cancer. People with high blood pressure, rheumatic heart disease or

overactive thyroids shouldn't supplement dietary
vitamin E without some medical supervision.

Vitamin C—Anti-aging, anti-stress, anti-viral, anti-
bacterial. Reduces serum cholesterol and (more
speculatively) helps prevent cancer, cavities, colds
and nosebleeds. Also protects the potency of other
vitamins.

Vitamin K—Helps promote good circulation and facilitates the clotting of wounds. The body usually
synthesizes its own supply of this vitamin without
any dietary supplementation.

MINERALS—THE GOOD GUYS

So far we have proteins and vitamins as the "good guys."

Fats, animal fats in particular, are the "bad guys."

And carbohydrates divide themselves on both teams, depending on whether or not man has deprived them of their natural
nutrition.

We have some important members still to come for the "good
guy" team—minerals.

But here we have another split. Some members of the
mineral team are outright poisons. One example is lead. It can
accumulate until it kills. I am going to list only the good guy
minerals and just what good they do,—the minerals essential to the
body:

Calcium—Forms and maintains bone hardness and
strength. Helps clot blood, transmit nerve impulses
and activate enzymes.

Phosphorous—A co-worker with calcium in the structur-
ing and maintenance of bones and teeth. Also
involved in the metabolism of fats and carbohydrates.

Magnesium—Steady nerves, carbohydrate metabolism.
A constitutent of bones and teeth.

Sulfur—Has protein-binding, energy-storing, poison
detoxifying properties.

> Sodium—Regulates nerve stability and muscular strength.
> Keeps body fluids in balance and flux. But can
> contribute to hypertension, causing problems.
> Potassium—Aside from doing everything sodium does
> from a slightly different perspective, potassium is
> also involved in the synthesis of protein and the
> maintaining of a regular heartbeat.
> Iodine—Helps regulate energy metabolsim.
> Iron—Helps bring oxygen to the blood and carbon
> dioxide away from the cells.
> Copper—Helps metabolize vitamin C and iron.
> Selenium—Anti-aging properties. Can stand in for Vita-
> min E but works best in conjunction with E and
> Vitamin C.

There is an important thing to remember about minerals.

You cannot get your iron from iron filings. A cold cereal manufacturer was recently caught inserting iron filings into the cereal and calling it fortified with iron. They would have done better using iron bars—at least the box would be strengthened.

We can use iron from spinach. We need plants and other animals to convert inorganic minerals for us into an organic form. Once so converted, the mineral can be metabolized.

Dolomite—in effect calcium made from pulverized calcium rock—does not help our bones one iota. In fact, it might even cause unwanted crystallization in our body, bone deposits, stones, etc. What helps our teeth and bones is organic calcium, like calcium lactate and pulverized oyster shells.

Now we are able to point to "wonder" foods that contain "good guy" nutrients. Wonder foods taste wonderful, but also do wonderful things for your health and longevity.

THE DIET PLAN: "WONDER" FOODS TO FAVOR
FOR LONGER LIFE

Nature provides us with everything we need to live out our natural span of years. Some say that Methuselah's nine hundred years is what we are all meant to live. Whatever the figure, it is certainly more than the 70 or 75 that we are managing to squeak out on the average.

And those extra years are supposed to be productive, enjoyable, active years, not nursing home years, invalid years, mentally incapacitated years, painful years.

Wonder foods can make the difference. There are probably a thousand or more on earth. But here, including the varieties within each category, we can number about one hundred. Look them over. Enjoy them on your Natural Protein Diet. And people will be looking you over.

Beef—lean cuts: Round steak, sirloin tip roast, cube steak, rump or English roast, flank steak, shank beef, porterhouse steak, tenderloin, lean stewing beef (trim excess fat off of all cuts). Veal—all types. Rich in protein, calcium, sodium, phosphorous, and sulfur. Good source of nucleic acids which are of possible longevity-promoting value. An average serving of beef or veal (3 1/2 oz.) provides 39-43% of your minimum daily protein needs.

Egg Whites: Fat-free, cholesterol-free portion of the egg. Rich in complete protein, potassium, sodium, sulfur and chlorine. An average serving of 1/2 oz. contains 21-25% of your minimum daily protein requirement.

Fish: High protein containing little or no carbohydrates and little fat. A 3 1/2 oz. serving of fish contains approximately 30-40% of your daily minimum protein needs. Most fish are rich in potassium, sodium, iodine, phosphorous, and sulfur and cell-building nucleic acids. Sardines are rich in protein, calcium and Vitamin D (needed to properly assimilate that calcium). Sardines are particularly high in nucleic acids (which may be of possible longevity-promoting value) which is good, but also in sodium a prime dietary contribution to hypertension and that's bad; so if you are on a low sodium diet eat them only occasionally. Eight medium sardines contain 32-39% of your minimum daily protein needs.

Poultry—Chicken and Turkey: Rich in complete protein (but low in fat), potassium, sulfur and phosphorous. Three slices of turkey provide 50-61% of your daily minimum protein needs. Chicken (breast)—35-42% your daily protein needs. The white meat has less fat than the dark.

Skim Milk: Excellent source of complete proteins, energizing milk sugars, phosphorous, sulfur and Vitamins A, B-complex and D (if suitably fortified by the manufacturer). One cup contains 16-20% of your daily minimum protein needs.

Buttermilk: Sour milk cultured with harmless bacteria. Buttermilk has a favorable effect on intestinal bacteria and is ideal for people allergic to ordinary milk. A favorite of the Abkhasians, long-lived people of Russia's Caucasus Mountain region, this lactic acid milk is a prime longevity promoting food. It does its work by helping to clear and revitalize cells clogged with metabolic debris. Buttermilk is cheaper in cost than yogurt and every bit as versatile. Use it as a salad dressing, dessert topping and in main dish sauces. One cup contains 16-20% of your daily minimum protein needs.

Yogurt (skim-milk variety): Defatted (96% fat free) milk fermented into a custard-like consistency and loaded with B-complex vitamins, calcium, phosphorous, sulfur, Vitamins A and D, and protein (in an instantly assimilable, predigested form). Yogurt is beneficial to digestion, intestinal health, the kidneys and is a natural antibiotic. Yogurt has been shown to have a cholesterol-lowering effect and is of possible value in treating arthritis, constipation, diarrhea, gallstones, halitosis, hepatitis, kidney disorders and skin diseases. Contains cell-revitalizing lactic acid and is a favorite of the long-lived Soviets, the Abkhasians. One cup contains 16-20% of your daily minimum protein needs. Read the label, especially of the new frozen varieties. Avoid those with chemical additives. Prefer those with natural flavors or plain.

Non-fat Dry Milk Solids: Excellent protein booster (also known as skim milk solids) for a wide variety of dishes or just plain milk. Non-fat dry milk solids contain about the same nutritional value as regular skim milk. 5 1/2 tablespoons provide 19-22% of your daily minimum protein needs.

Acidophilus Milk: A soured milk available in health food stores and similar to yogurt and buttermilk in most nutritional and health promoting properties. Acidophilus milk aids and assists the digestive system by helping to establish beneficial bacteria in the intestine and soothing digestive tract inflammations.

Cottage Cheese (low fat variety): Especially rich in complete milk proteins and an excellent source of calcium, phosphorous and sulfur. Six tablespoons (3 1/2 oz.) of uncreamed cottage cheese contains 26-31% of your daily minimum protein needs.

Farmer's Cheese: A very nutritious low-fat cheese, rich in protein, calcium, potassium, phosphorous and sulfur. An average serving provides 6-7% of your daily minimum protein needs.

Cheddar and Swiss Cheeses: Of all the cheeses these two are particularly rich in bone-building, nerve soothing calcium. They are also rich in protein, phosphorous and sulfur. Since they are not as low in fat as some cheeses, cheddar and swiss should only be eaten occasionally. One ounce of either cheese provides 12-14% of your daily minimum protein needs.

Low-fat Cheeses (skim milk ricotta, skim milk mozzarella): Rich in protein, calcium, potassium, phosphorous and sulfur. An average serving provides about 12-14% of your daily minimum protein needs.

Rye Bread: A whole-grain bread, rich in incomplete protein (of a higher quality than either white or whole wheat bread), oil, starches, potassium, phosphorous and sulfur. One slice provides 2-3% of your daily minimum protein needs.

Whole Wheat Bread: Rich in incomplete protein, wheat germ oil and carbohydrates. Good source of phosphorous, potassium, sulfur and Vitamin E. Whole wheat bread is generally beneficial to digestive health and is a favorite of long-lived peoples around the world. One slice contains 2-3% of your daily minimum protein needs.

Wheat Bran: Highly beneficial digestive bulk food that helps prevent diverticulosis, polyps, colitis, hemmorhoids and cancer of the rectum and colon. Two round tablespoons provides 2-3% of your daily minimum protein requirement.

Wheat Germ: The heart of whole wheat, a kernel; rich in Vitamin E, B-complex and iron. Also contains good to fair amounts of copper, magnesium, manganese, calcium and phosphorous. High in nucleic acids, which are of possible longevity-promoting value. Only two tablespoons provide 5-6% of your daily minimum protein needs. Wheat germ is delicious sprinkled on cereals or baked into meat loaves. Since it is highly perishable, wheat germ should be refrigerated after opening. An interesting but underlying benefit of wheat germ is its role as an anti-stress factor. Any condition that causes damage to the body is stress, whether it is derived from overwork, bacterial invasion or insufficiencies in diet or sleep. Wheat germ contains vital anit-stress ingredients which create a marked resistance to various bacteria. The greater the stress level of the individual the more susceptible he is to both the initial onset of illness and to its potential severity.

Triticale: A wonder grain of the future, not generally available now outside of health food stores. Triticale (trit-i-kay-lee) is a hybrid combination of wheat and rye flours with 40% more protein potency together than either has individually. Triticale is delicious sprinkled on cereals or baked into homemade breads. One-third cup provides 14-17% of your daily minimum protein needs.

Buckwheat: A cereal grain available in supermarkets as groats or kasha (medium or coarse). Buckwheat is rich in potassium, phosphorous and sulfur. Buckwheat is also an excellent source of rutin, an anti-allergy substance beneficial to the health of your respiratory and circulatory system in general. An average serving of buckwheat provides 12-14% of your daily minimum protein needs.

Sourdough Bread: Comparable in nutritional value to most other breads but with the added bonuses of containing longevity-promoting lactic acid and no health-harming shortening (vegetable or otherwise).

Shredded Wheat: Popular nutritious breakfast cereal with none of the health-harming additives of most other kinds, but plenty of natural fiber and bulk to assist digestion and aid your intestinal tract. One biscuit of shredded wheat contains 7-8% of your daily minimum protein needs. Remember, most grains are incomplete protein but by including several on your menu, one may provide what the other is lacking.

Brown Rice: A high-powered B-complex grain and a good source of calcium, phosphorous and iron. It is a whole-grain food;

contains cholesterol reducing bran and some oil (and because of that oil, brown rice should be refrigerated after opening to maintain optimum freshness). One-third cup of brown rice contains 7-8% of your daily minimum protein needs.

Wild Rice: Rich in incomplete protein and with the sole exception of calcium, contains more mineral elements (iron, magnesium, potassium, phosphorous and zinc) than brown rice or polished white rice. Also an excellent source of Vitamins B-1, B-2 and niacin. Contains 14-16% of your minimum daily protein needs per 1/3 cup.

Birchermuesli: A nutritious Swiss breakfast cereal available in health food stores and supermarkets under the brand names of Alpen, Swiss Familia and others. Birchermuesli generally contains wheat, raw oatmeal flakes, barley, dried fruits (currants or small raisins), nuts (raw hazelnuts, filberts or almonds) and wheat germ. Birchermuesli also comes in a candy bar form available in health food stores.

Oats (oatmeal): A rich source of incomplete protein, potassium, phosphorous, sulfur and silicon. Oats are a good source of nucleic acids (DNA and RNA) which are concentrated cell nutrients of possible use in promoting longevity. Oats have been shown to be of value in reducing serum cholesterol. They also provide much needed bulk and fiber for the health of the digestive tract. One-third cup of oats provides 7-8% of your daily minimum protein needs.

Pastas: Soy, artichoke, whole wheat or buckwheat noodles are varieties generally available in health food stores and loaded with nutritional value instead of the empty calories of most other brands. Plain, ordinary pasta:—a life shortener. These other pastas: —life extenders.

Asparagus: Very rich in the amino acid known as asparagine and Vitamin A. Asparagus is also a good source of nucleic acids and substances called histones, which are currently being investigated for cancer preventative properties. Five to six spears of asparagus contain 5-6% of your daily minimum protein requirement.

Brussel Sprouts: Miniature cabbages containing a rich supply of incomplete plant protein, cholesterol—controlling cellulose, potassium, phosphorous and sulfur. Nine medium-sized brussel sprouts contain 7-8% of your daily minimum protein needs.

Squash: Rich source of the longevity-promoting B-complex, anti-infective Vitamin A and minerals (especially potassium).

Corn: A nutritious whole grain source of incomplete protein and Vitamin B-1 (thiamine) and A. Corn is especially noted for its rich methionine (one of the eight essential amino acids) content. Methionine is beneficial to the health of the skin and scalp and helps promote liver health. 3 1/2 oz. of corn provides approximately 7-8% of your daily minimum protein needs.

Tomato: A delicious fruit (a berry usually included in the diet as a "vegetable") rich in Vitamin C and A. The tomato is also a good source of B-2 (and other B-complex vitamins) and the nerve-soothing, heartprotecting mineral element, potassium.

Jerusalem Artichoke (not Globe or French kind): A root vegetable related to sunflower seeds and a rich source of minerals (iron and phosphorous) and a carbohydrate called inulin, which (lucky for dieters) is not absorbed by the body. Jerusalem artichokes can be used in place of potatoes by those on a reducing diet and is often recommended by doctors as being suitable eating fare for diabetics.

Endive (also known as chicory): Very rich in Vitamin A (one of the three highest vegetable sources) and potassium. Endive is a natural aid to regular elimination and indigestion, also believed to be of help in alleviating some liver troubles.

"Calorie-less" foods: Beans, green or wax; bean sprouts, turnips, cauliflower, cucumbers, mushrooms, peppers, pimentos, summer squash and eggplant. As a group, "calorie-less" foods aren't much on vitamins (except for Vitamin A) but they are big on roughage and you can pretty much eat your fill of that without putting on a pound (which is a blessing in and of itself). Turnips and cauliflower are favorites of the long-lived Hunzas. Spinach, dandelion greens, and turnip greens are "sleepers" in our vegetable bins. Buy them whenever available—fresh is better than frozen, frozen is better than not at all.

Kale: Cabbage leaves by any other name and an excellent source of Vitamin A (along with parsley and escarole, kale is one of the three highest vegetable sources of this vitamin), B-complex and C. Kale also contains a good to fair supply of potassium, calcium, iron, phosphorous and sodium. 3/4 cup contains 5-6% of your daily minimum protein needs.

Okra: A rich source of incomplete vegetable protein (low in carbohydrates, no fat), sodium and calcium. Okra is a beneficial aid for digestion and is of assistance in soothing inflammations of the stomach and intestines (such as ulcers and colitis).

Broccoli: A nutritious vegetable rich in potassium, Vitamin-B-complex and Vitamin C. Has been known to be of use in alleviating the symptoms of migraine sufferers.

Pumpkin: Good source of anti-infective Vitamin A; cholesterol-controlling cellulose and pectin, the longevity-promoting B-complex and anti-aging Vitamin C. Don't buy it in a can as for pie filling. You'll be fooling yourself.

Sweet Potato: An excellent source of calcium and phosphorous. Sweet potatoes also contain a healthy amount of anti-infective, anti-aging Vitamin A.

Sauerkraut: White cabbage that has been allowed to ferment in longevity, promoting lactic acid. Sauerkraut is rich in potassium and calcium and Vitamin A, D, and C. It is a favorite of the long-lived Soviet Abkhasians.

Alfalfa: Nutritious vegetable food available in supermarkets as sprouts for salads. Alfalfa is one of the richest sources of vitamins and minerals. Alfalfa contains ten different vitamins and at least eight natural enzymes deemed beneficial for digestive health. Rich in vitamins A, C, and D and B-2 and very high in calcium and iron, alfalfa is often praised as being one of the most complete foods there is. Later, I'll tell you how to grow sprouts in your kitchen and save money.

Green Beans: Otherwise known as string beans. Not spectacular eating fare but it has virtually no calories and contains a fair percentage of all the vitamins, and that's a small blessing for the conscientious "live longer" fan.

An interesting but distressing statistic is the increase of ill health parallelling the sales and consumption of refined foods, sugared cereals, soft drinks and "snacks," with the decreased use of vegetables. Over and over again I have been informed by children, teenagers and people in their mid-years that they "hate" vegetables (with the exception of french fries) and are unable to name one which they enjoy. In almost every case they remember as a child being forced to taste or eat vegetables because "they are good for you." Coincidentally, most of the non-vegetable eaters are now overweight. School kitchens report that over 60% of children receiving hot lunches do not touch their green vegetables (they will, however, eat mashed potatotes if covered with gravy, preferably thick and sticky). It is a sad commentary that a healthy source of potassium and many other minerals and vitamins find their way only too often to the garbage can.

Lentils: A nutritious legume (other "legumes" are peas and beans), rich in plant protein, cellulose, potassium, sodium, calcium, phosphorous, sulfur and nucleic acids. Lentils are reported to have beneficial anti-toxic properties and to be of use in treating anemia, dyspepsia and inflammation of the intestine.

Peas (fresh, green): Rich source of vegetable protein and energy-promoting carbohydrates. Peas are also rich in magnesium, potassium, phosphorous, sulfur and nucleic acids, with goodly amounts of Vitamins A, C, B-1 and B-2 as well. A 3/4 cup of fresh green peas contains 7-8% of your daily minimum protein allowance.

Chick Peas: Also known as garbonzos, nahit (in Yiddish), and chana dal (in Hindu), chick peas are an undervalued and under-appreciated legume that gives as much protein in an average serving as 4 1/2 ounces of steak. Chick peas are rich in heart-protecting potassium, cholesterol-reducing phytosterols, strength-promoting iron and bone-building calcium. Chick peas also contain good amounts of niacin, thiamine (B-1) and riboflavin (B-2). A 1/4 -1/3 cup serving contains 12-14% of your minimum daily protein requirement. Chick peas are a favorite food of the long-lived Hunzas.

Mung Beans: Rich in plant proteins, B-complex vitamins and nucleic acids. 1/4-1/3 cup of mung beans provides 16-20% of your daily minimum protein needs. Good to sprout, also.

Lima Beans: A good source of incomplete protein and the kind of carbohydrate that is more effective than bran in lowering serum cholesterol and firming the intestinal tract. Lima beans are also good source of nucleic acids and energy-promoting substances known as purines. A 1/2 cup portion provides 9-11% of your daily minimum protein needs. Somewhat high in calories.

Onions: Raw onions are a rich source of anti-aging Vitamin C, strength-promoting iron, nerve-soothing potassium and bone-building calcium. Onions are well-known appetite stimulants.

Green Peppers: Primarily a top-notch flavoring addition to salads and stews, green peppers are also an excellent source of anti-infective Vitamins A and C.

Chives: A rich source of incomplete protein, oil, calcium and potassium. This onion-type vegetable is also an excellent flavoring aid and digestive stimulant.

Garlic: An excellent source of raw fiber (a digestive aid), potassium, calcium, phosphorous, Vitamin A, B-complex and Vitamin C. Garlic stimulates the appetite and digestive secretions and helps heal inflammations of the intestines brought on by constipation. Garlic has been known to help control high blood pressure and respiratory troubles. Rich in antibiotic phytoncides, garlic is particularly effective against intestinal parasites.

Raw Juices: Easy to digest, body regenerators and rejuvenators. *Raw carrot juice* is very rich in Vitamin A with plenty of Vitamin B, C, D, E and K as well. *Apple juice* aids digestion. *Celery juice* is a potent nerve tonic. *Cucumber juice* infuses minerals into our systems that are beneficial to hair growth. *Brussel sprout juice* provides a natural sugar-digesting insulin to aid our own. *Onion juice* helps kill health-endangering bacteria in the nose and throat.

Raw Foods: Grains, vegetables, fruits, seeds, nuts, juices and oils. Raw foods are notably rich in auxones, vitamin-enzymatic substances highly necessary to the promotion of health and longevity.

Apple: Rich in fruit-acid salts which help aid digestive processes and pectin which helps control serum cholesterol. Pectin also counteracts the toxic effects of numerous drugs, chemicals and food additives and is known to help protect the body from radiation damage. Uncooked and unpeeled apples contain some Vitamin E.

Grape: Rich in digestion-aiding fruit-acid salts, natural energizing sugars, potassium, B-complex and Vitamin C. Purple or red grapes contain virus-killing polyphenols that can go to work in your digestive system as a natural antibiotic and antiseptic. Grapes also lessen the formation of harmful uric acids in the body and contribute towards more regular elimination.

Orange: Rich in digestion-aiding fruit, acid salts, calcium, potassium and Vitamins A, C, and B-complex. One medium-sized orange contains 200% of your daily minimum requirement of Vitamin C.

Tangerine: One large tangerine contains about 90% of your daily minimum allowance of Vitamin C.

Grapefruit: Rich in Vitamin A, calcium, iron, magnesium, phosphorous, potassium and Vitamin C. (200% of your recommended daily allowance.)

Peaches: An excellent source of anti-aging, anti-infective Vitamin A, bone-building calcium and heart-protecting potassium. Peaches help relieve constipation and aid the digestive process in general. Three medium-sized peaches contain over 90% of your minimum daily requirement for Vitamin A.

Papaya: A delicious fruit, rich in incomplete protein, low in fat, and high in natural energizing sugars. Good source of magnesium, phosphorous, sulfur, Vitamin A, Vitamin C and the B-complex. Known as the "magical melon of the tropics," papaya is rich in papain, an excellent protein-digesting enzyme and natural digestive aid. In growing availability from Puerto Rico and Hawaii.

Avocado: A no-starch, low sugar fruit, rich in potassium, Vitamin A and highly digestible oils. Avocado is known to assist elimination, control serum cholesterol and stimulate appetite.

Blackberry: A rich source of natural energizing sugars and cholesterol-controlling cellulose. A tea made from the blackberry's leaves, fruit and roots is believed to be beneficial to controlling diarrhea and digestive trace inflammations.

Plum: Very rich in fruit sugars and potassium. Plums also contain a fair amount of digestion-aiding fruit acid salts. They assist in the relief of constipation and hemorrhoids. Plums beneficially stimulate the intestinal tract and in that regard have been used to assist the treatment of liver ailments.

Pineapple: Rich in potassium, cholesterol-controlling cellulose and (in uncooked state only) protein-digesting papain. Pineapples are known to facilitate proper digestion by supplying the stomach with natural acid salts.

Apricot: The favorite fruit of the long-lived Hunzas who claim that a good deal of their fabled health and longevity is due to its nutritional goodness. Apricots are rich in potassium and iron and especially rich in longevity-promoting Vitamin A. Five medium-sized apricots contain 100% of your daily minimum Vitamin A needs. Remember, dried fruits go a long way. Enjoy them moderately—they are high in calories.

Cherry: Rich in natural energizing sugars, digestion-aiding fruit acids and nerve-soothing potassium. Cherries are also an excellent source of anti-aging Vitamins C and B-complex. Taken on a daily basis, cherries tend to benefit regular elimination and your health in general.

Strawberry: Rich in fruit sugars and natural bacteriacides that promote better digestive health. Strawberries are also a good source of anti-aging, anti-infective Vitamin C.

Mango: Tropical fruit, rich in energizing sugars and Vitamins A and C. One mango provides half of your minimum Vitamin A needs and all of your daily Vitamin C needs. The mango is more expensive than most fruits and harder to come by, but well worth having for variety as well as nutrition in your daily diet. Natural to our 50th State, Hawaii.

Kiwi Fruit: From New Zealand and loaded with plenty of anti-aging, anti-infective Vitamin C. The "Kiwi" is a tasty treat with a strawberry-watermelon type flavor.

Wheat Germ Oil: A thick amber oil available in liquid form or capsules in health food stores and some drugstores and supermarkets. Wheat germ oil is your best source of heart-protecting, anti-aging Vitamin E outside of taking the isolated vitamin itself. One tablespoon provides 100% of your daily minimum requirement for Vitamin E. Wheat germ oil has been found to be of significant value in fighting fatigue and increasing endurance in athletes and others. Wheat germ oil is fine on salads or can be taken mixed with a glass of milk or carrot juice. This largely polyunsaturated oil is highly subject to rancidity, so keep it refrigerated after opening to preserve its freshness and potency.

Peanuts: Excellent source of protein (incomplete), potassium, calcium, magnesium, phosphorous and sulfur. Two tablespoons provide 7-8% of your daily minimum protein needs.

Cashew Nuts: Rich in protein, iron and Vitamins B-1 and D. 12-16 nuts provide 7-8% of your daily minimum protein needs.

Sesame Seeds: Top-notch source of protein, cholesterol-controlling lecithin and polyunsaturated oils, Vitamins B-complex and E, and calcium and phosphorous. Three tablespoons of sesame seeds contain 7-8% of your daily minimum protein needs.

Soybeans: Rich in complete, highly digestible plant protein, heart-protecting vegetable fat, calcium, phosphorous, potassium, magnesium and iron. Soybeans are also a good source of Vitamin B-complex, Vitamin A, Vitamin E and a cholesterol-controlling substance called lecithin. 1/4 - 1/3 cup of soybeans provides 23-28% of your complete minimum protein needs.

Black Walnuts: (not English Walnuts which are high in calories and qualitatively low in protein): Rich in incomplete protein and unsaturated fats. Black walnuts contain some calcium and fair quantities of potassium, magnesium, phosphorous and sulfur. They are a good source of nucleic acids and a favorite of the long-lived Soviets, the Abkhasians. Some 16 to 20 black walnut halves contain 7-8% of your daily minimum protein needs.

Sunflower Seeds: A good source of iron, phosphorous, calcium, iodine, magnesium, potassium, manganese, copper, Vitamins B-1, B-2, niacin, B-6, para-amino-benzoic acid, and Vitamins

D and E. Sunflower seeds are rich in protein, unsaturated fats and fiber and pectin which are highly beneficial to stamina and heart and nerve health. High in nucleic acids. Three tablespoons of sunflower seeds contain 9-11% of your daily minimum protein needs.

Pumpkin Seeds: Rich in Vitamin A, phosphorous, iron, and unsaturated oils. Raw pumpkin seeds contain a hormone material reputed to be of help in treating male prostate troubles. Pumpkin seeds should be eaten raw and unsalted in order for you to obtain their full nutritional value. Two tablespoons supply 12-14% of your daily minimum protein needs.

Apple-Cider Vinegar: A liquid derived from fresh and aged apples used as a healthful salad dressing, quick thirst quencher (when mixed with water) or as an excellent skin tonic. Apple-cider vinegar is a good source of vitamins, minerals and highly beneficial digestive enzymes.

Acerola Cherries: A tropical fruit and one of the richest known sources of Vitamin C. One cherry contains 100% of your recommended daily requirement of Vitamin C. Acerola cherries are available in health foods in juice concentrate, powder, tablet or capsule form.

Camu-Camu: A tangerine-flavored plum-like tropical fruit exceedingly rich in Vitamin C. Camu-camu is available in health food stores as a delicious table concentrate.

Rose Hips: Supplementary food available in health food stores in a variety of forms (tablets, capsules, powders, syrups, jams, jellies, candies and teas). Rose hips are the Vitamin C rich seed pods or fruit of the rose flower. One tablespoon of liquid rose hips contain an incredible 400% of your daily minimum requirement of Vitamin C.

Pollen: Available in health food stores, pollen is one of the richest sources of concentrated food nutrients there is. A fermented substance from fruit or vegetable plants, pollen is collected from honeycombs and then processed into granules or tablets loaded with amino acids, vitamins and minerals. Pollen is rich in natural antibiotics and bactericides that help maintain intestinal health. Pollen is 35% protein, half of which is in instantly assimilable (requires no enzymatic digestion) amino acids. Pollen is a standard part of many long-lived peoples' diets.

Amino Acid Compounds: Highly digestible and assimilable liquid protein available as a dietary aid in health food stores and some drug stores. An excellent way to occasionally supplement the protein in your daily diet, amino acid compounds can be taken with milk, juice or various vegetable juices. Do not use as a weight loss diet unless under the supervision of your physician.

Brewer's Yeast: A powerhouse of nutrition, brewer's yeast contains 16 amino acids, 14 minerals and 17 vitamins and a little or a lot of just about every known nutrient (exceptions are Vitamins B-12, A, C, and E). Brewer's yeast is an excellent source of complete (almost pure) protein (no starch, no fat), Vitamins B-1, B-2, B-6, niacin, choline, inusitol, pantothenic acid, para-aminobenzoic acid, amino acids, lysine, tryptophane, histidine, phenylalanine, leucine, methionine, valine, glycine, alanine, aspartic acid, glutamic acid, proline, hydroxproline, tyrosin, cystine, arginine, minerals — phosphorous, potassium, magnesium, silicon, calcium, copper, manganese zinc, aluminum, sodium, iron, tin, boron, gold, silver, nickel, cobalt, iodine and nucleic acids. Experimental evidence has shown brewer's yeast to be of possible value in treating some cancer, hepatits, senile dementia, constipation and heart troubles. Brewer's yeast is especially rich in the three B vitamins (B-6, folic acid, pantothenic acid) needed to produce infection-fighting antibodies. Brewer's yeast can be added to vegetable or fruit juices or baked into meat loaves, hashes, soups and stuffings. One level tablespoon contains 5-6% of your minimum daily protein requirement.

A friend of mine who is a nutritionist at an experimental nutritional center in Toronto, Canada, tells me of the use of brewers yeast taken directly from a brewery after it had been used in the manufacture of beer. The clinic uses this product with success in lowering blood cholesterol in many patients. An alcoholic ward of a municipal hospital has found this substance of remarkable value in conditions of cirrhosis of the liver. Further benefits were obtained in radical cases of eczema and presently there is experimentation in the control of growth of gallstones and in the control of nausea derived from radiation therapy. Many people who add brewers yeast to their diet speak happily about their increased energy. In one particular case a factory worker who worked with dangerous equipment had to discontinue that type of work because by midday he became too tired to concentrate. The addition of brewer's yeast to his diet enabled him to complete his work without the fatigue that he formerly suffered.

Dessicated Liver: A concentrated form of beef liver available in powder or tablet form in health food stores and some drug stores. Dessicated liver is an excellent source of Vitamin A, B-complex, copper, calcium and concentrated protein. Dessicated liver is notably rich in the "youth vitamin" pantothenic acid. One tablespoon supplies approximately 10% of your daily minimum protein needs. Dessicated liver can be mixed with hamburger meat, vegetable juices, soups and stews.

Bone Meal: Powdered beef bones available in health food stores. Bone meal is an extremely rich source of bone building calcium and phosphorous in concentrated form.

Carob: A delicious substitute for chocolate with almost the exact same taste and none of chocolate's allergy-promoting or nerve-irritating properties. Carob is rich in potassium, calcium and phosphorous. Carob is known to be a beneficial aid for regular elimination. It is available in tablet, powder, syrup and candy-bar-wafer form.

Blackstrap Molasses: Powder-packed sweetener available in health food stores. Rich in calcium (proportionately more than milk), copper, magnesium, phosphorous, pantothenic acid, inositol and Vitamin E. Also a particularly excellent source of iron and all the B-complex vitamins. Blackstrap molasses is of possible value in alleviating a wide variety of ailments from anemia to constipation. Blackstrap molasses is a derivative of cane sugar and as such sticks to your teeth with an especially powerful decay-promoting vengeance—so it is recommended that you brush your teeth immediately after using it.

Lecithin: A fatty substance found in every part of the human body. Lecithin is considered vital to proper cellular function (though no minimum daily requirement has yet been set) and of possible longevity—promoting value when eaten in sufficient amounts. Found naturally in egg yolk, soybeans and corn, lecithin has been known to reduce serum cholesterol, to lower blood pressure (in some people), and to alleviate symptoms of eczema, acne and psoriasis. Lecithin also helps the body assimilate Vitamins A and E and helps prevent deposits of fat in the liver and blood stream. Besides being obtainable from dietary sources lecithin is also available in capsule, tablet, powder, liquid or granular form in health food stores and some drug stores.

Mineral Water: Plain pure water without lime and other health-harming impurities. An excellent brand available at health food stores is Ramlosa, bottled at the famous European spa at Ramlosabrunn.

Well, there you have the "wonder" foods that I recommend. Note, I have included protein percentages and whether complete or incomplete. In the next chapter, I tell you how to build your own Natural Protein Diet.

Chapter 4

Your Food Selection
for the Petrie Protein Diet

Do not see yourself eating a breakfast of figs, a lunch of yogurt and a dinner of turnip greens. This is not the Petrie Diet.

What then is the Diet? It is just what you are eating now with a few substitutions. We will drop empty calories and substitute calories that are brimming with nutrition. We will drop fat calories and substitute low-fat calories. Both of these substitutions are in the direction of higher protein.

The reason my clients look younger on this diet is because the body responds to vitamins, minerals and protein, especially when they arrive in place of white bread, greasy bacon, and fudge.

Research is going on in expanding circles. There is the American Geriatrics Society, 10 Columbus Circle, New York City, founded back in 1942. Its 8,000 members include physicians, physiotherapists, occupational therapists, social and welfare workers including a few superintendents of hospitals and homes for the aged. The staff of five is charged with encouraging and promoting the study of geriatrics and stressing the importance of medical research in the field of aging.

Would you prefer to wait for meaningful findings to be announced? Or would you prefer to start your youthing process today?

There is also the Aging Research Institute at 342 Madison Avenue, New York, which does excellent work, I am sure, in supporting research into the aging process in man, including studies of the embryonic, mature and aging cells in all their phases and research in the prevention, diagnosis and treatment of diseases of advancing years.

Would you prefer to age and hope that research will ease the symptoms? Or would you like to prolong your youth as much as possible, starting now?

There is also the American Aging Association, founded in 1970 at the University of Nebraska College of Medicine, dedicated to helping people live longer by promoting bio-medical aging studies directed at slowing down the aging process and increasing the knowledge of this among physicians and other health workers.

And there is the Gerontological Society, 1 Dupont Circle, Washington, D. C., with 4,000 members, most of them professional researchers in the behavioral, social, and biological sciences with two publications: *The Gerontologist* and *Journal of Gerontology*. And don't forget the Association for Advancement of Aging Research, 309 Hancock Building, University of Southern California, Los Angeles and the National Geriatrics Society, 212 Wisconsin Avenue in Milwaukee, Wisconsin.

There are probably more in the country that I have not heard of and many more in Europe, Asia, and throughout the world.

All are doing spendid work and breakthroughs are occurring. I have supplied the addresses in case you would like to investigate further.

But while waiting for a reply, and while "hanging in" there until practical actions are available for your extended life, would you like to extend your life nutritionally in the only way known to man—starting today?

It is easy. It is fun. It is rewarding. It is the only sure way you have to beat the odds.

Did I hear you say, "Yes!"? How young your voice sounds.

TO EAT CORRECTLY AND LIVE LONGER
OR TO EAT INCORRECTLY AND DIE SOONER

In 1975, Americans smoked 600 billion cigarettes. Each smoker forfeited up to five or more minutes of life with each cigarette. That adds up to an aggregate of five million years of life voluntarily lost by Americans that year, just by smoking.

There is no way to add up the years lost by fat-rich foods and empty sweets and starches, but I'll wager it far exceeds the years of life lost through smoking. More people eat than smoke, and eating can be just as fatal as smoking.

These years of life lost through eating are also voluntary.

We have the choice: to eat correctly or not. Yet, so many of us eaters seem to have the same devil-may-care attitude as do the smokers. It is as if there was a death wish lurking in most of us, especially in that fat man over there, sitting at the counter and having apple pie a la mode and in that young couple over there, sharing a banana split and in that hefty woman over there, carrying potato chips with her.

If it is a subliminal death wish that drives us to these killing foods, we certainly don't recognize it as such. In fact, quite the contrary. We dive into the pies, sweets, and chips as though our lives depended on it.

A smoker also lights up as though his life depended on it. That first inhalation of smoke is treated as if it was the first breath of fresh air after days of entombment. The person out of cigarettes will walk a mile for any brand.

You answered "yes" to my question a moment ago. How do you answer to this question: Do you have a death wish?

Of course, you have answered no. Yet you, too, are guilty of plunging into death-dealing foods. Why?

Well, I have news for you. . .

You have been manipulated.

It is not your fault really. You have read the ads. You have seen the food packages. You have listened to the commercials. You bought. You prepared. You tasted. It was quick and easy. It tasted good. You bought again.

The food manufacturing and packaging industries have done a good job. Supermarkets now offer a great variety of choices compared to old grocery store, meat market, and fish market. The country food stores—the mom and pop stores that handled mostly local produce—are out of business.

Produce now travels hundreds of miles, maybe thousands. It is picked or harvested before it is ripe in order to travel that distance without spoiling. Colorants are placed on fruits to compensate for the resulting poor coloring.

You buy what is available. You buy what is reasonable. You buy what is easy to prepare.

The food producers have exploited these human needs to provide products that are in more variety, reasonable and easy to prepare, usually at the expense of your nutrition.

So you have acquired eating habits that include useless foods. You may gain weight but you lose years.

It is not easy to get out of the danish pastry habit or the ice cream habit. But people are doing so every day.

It comes about easier when you substitute even better foods in their place. But the process takes coaxing on your part until a new habit is formed.

I promise you will have the new habit longer than the old. Because you will live longer as a result of it.

THE BASIC LONGEVITY DIET GUIDELINES

Here is the basic outline of my longevity diet. It is the structure on which you will hang the specific nutritional foods that you yourself select.

You might call these the *LONGEVITY DIET GUIDELINES:*

MEAT:	Choose from lean cuts. Veal is always lean; use any cut of veal. Avoid smoked meats like sausage, frankfurters, cold cuts.
POULTRY:	Chicken or turkey, white meat preferably. Remove all visible fats from meat and the skin from poultry.
FISH:	All types.
EGGS:	Only two eggs yolks may be eaten weekly. However, egg whites may be used at will.
FRUITS:	All fruits may be used but sugar-packed fruits or fruits in syrup must be avoided. People with a weight problem should avoid dried fruits.
VEGETABLES:	All may be used.

BREAD:	Should be made of sourdough and baked without shortening or sugar. But an occasional slice of whole wheat or rye bread is allowed.
RICE, PASTA, NOODLES:	Allowable but avoid if made with eggs.
CEREAL:	Allowable but avoid if made with shortening or sugar.
MILK:	Use low fat only.
CHEESE:	Only if made from low fat milk.
FATS, OILS:	Maximum one tablespoon daily.
SOUPS:	Allowable if made from any ingredients contained in the diet.
BEVERAGES:	Water, plain soda water, vegetable or unsweetened fruit juices, dry wine, tea, coffee (maximum 6 oz. daily).

As you examine the above categories, you see immediately that you can eat practically everything on the Longevity Diet. Nothing important is eliminated. However, some foods high in fat or carbohydrates are curtailed in quantity and some are changed in quality.

It is better for your body if you enjoy the breast of chicken instead of the thighs.

It is better for your body if you enjoy sourdough or whole wheat bread instead of plain white bread.

It is better for your body if you enjoy pot cheese and cottage cheese more than Swiss cheese and American cheese.

How much better? It is impossible to relate one slice of white bread to minutes or seconds of life lost as a cigarette has been equated to five minutes.

The greatest variable in making such determinations are people. Some centenarians have eaten white bread much of their lives. Other old people have doted on fatty or starchy foods and lived to brag about it.

But how do you know you are such a person? It would be fool-hardy to add white bread to your longevity diet on the chance you are going to die for some other reason. "It can't happen to me" says the smoker. And, similarly, millions of Americans are playing Russian roulette with pizza, pastry, and pie.

If there is something not allowed on this diet, find a way around it, rather than take a chance with those added years. I'll be helping you to do this with menus and recipes, with new foods you may have never tried, to replace the old—in you.

HOW TO DEAL WITH YOUR EXTRA POUNDS ON THE LONGEVITY DIET

Agnes A., 36, taught special classes for emotionally disturbed children. She had been gradually gaining weight over ten years and had tried various diets. At 230 pounds she began to suffer from ulcers and decided to include some "wonder" foods in her diet for better health.

She still was seriously bothered by her ulcers and had to be hospitalized. There she was put on a bland diet of milk and cream. Her weight kept climbing. She began to have periods of severe depression and anxiety. She was in a state of perpetual fatigue, with or without "wonder" foods. Her work suffered and she saw it was just a matter of time before she would have to quit her job.

That was when she came to my office. She agreed with me that, if good physical and mental health was her objective, the pounds would have to come off first. I took her off the few "wonder" foods she was eating and put her on a low carbohydrate, low fat diet. That meant high in protein. I discussed this with her physician so that we were able to include the necessary milk therapy for the ulcerous condition.

It took some reconditioning. Agnes had been eating quickie foods like cakes and pastries. I showed her an easy way to stop,— the same mental reprogramming techniques that I will tell you how to use later. It enables you to shift from unwanted "habit" foods easily, without willpower.

Agnes lost 53 pounds in two months. Then her progress chart flattened out. She was feeling so much better that she realized more than ever before the big difference those excess pounds made in her health. "How can I continue to lose?" she asked.

I explained that she had another habit she needed to cope with. She was still serving herself the same portions despite the fact that her body had shrunk by about 20 percent. We used the same reconditioning technique to make smaller portions normal for her.

Agnes' weight tumbled again. She reached her goal of 160 and set a new goal of 135. She gained new energy. In fact, she became a dynamo in the community, joining a swimming club, becoming active in a civic organization, and always socially in demand.

Her ulcers? It turned out they were not "hers" after all. No more stomach trouble. No more depression. No more fatigue. All without "wonder" foods. She was then able to return to seeds (her favorite) and whole grains without irritating her sensitive stomach lining. Her appearance was vastly improved by the loss of weight, but the "wonder" foods gave her a youthful radiance. She glowed with health, looking and feeling years younger.

If you are overweight you need to give top priority to this problem.

If you are 35 or 40 years old and you are thinking about longevity while you have been 25 to 50 percent overweight for a number of years, you are slated to live 20 to 30 years less, not more.

The actuarial tables show that a man, 35, who should weigh 150 but who has weighed 250 for most of his adult years can expect to live 28 years less than if he was normal weight.

A woman, 35, who has been only 25 percent overweight most of her adult years, weighing 150 instead of 120 is taking seven years off her life expectancy.

So you can equate extra pounds to years lost, and pounds lost to years gained.

The Longevity Diet can be shaped to meet the needs of many different tastes and food requirements, but if your shape is oval that is what needs to shape your Longevity Diet.

In Chapter 8 you will find how to create menus that supply top noursihment to your body while fat melts away.

If you are overweight, this is your top priority chapter, and you are in for a double reward,—the rejuvenation that comes with dropping "excess baggage," and then the vigorous health that comes with the "wonder" foods.

COMBINING FOODS FOR A BALANCED DIET

Whether or not you go on a weight loss diet first, your daily intake must be a balanced one.

Where health problems have arisen because of a diet, it has usually been because of one extreme or another. Extremely low quantity can starve the vital organs. They can literally consume themselves. Extremes in types of food, like mostly rice or mostly grapefruit or mostly steak can still starve the body of some mineral or vitamin needed for normal functioning.

The balanced diet is the only way to diet. Weight loss, longevity, both—a proper proportion of different foods needs to be part of the daily fare.

Here is a table that provides guidelines for balancing your diet. I will explain the quantities listed as portions, but first examine the table.

IDEAL BALANCE OF DAILY FOODS IN LONGEVITY DIET

BEEF:	3 ounces daily (cooked weight)
or	
POULTRY, FISH:	6 ounces daily (cooked weight)
EGGS:	One or two egg whites daily
FRUITS:	4 ounces daily
VEGETABLES:	6 ounces daily
BREAD:	1 or 2 slices daily
RICE, PASTA, NOODLES:	Choose from one portion daily (3 ounces)
CEREAL:	One portion daily
MILK:	One 8 ounce glass daily
CHEESE:	Two ounces daily

Total calorie count on above intake—1,400 calories.

This to most people would be a reducing diet. To adjust upwards consult the abbreviated calorie count table in Chapter 8. You can safely increase the calorie count to 2,000 or more daily if weight reduction is not your problem.

How do you add to the above quantities and still keep a balanced diet? A 50 percent across the board increase in the portions would be the approach for translation to a non-weight loss basis.

This would give you a balanced diet of about 2,000 calories. The average person will not gain weight on a balanced 2,000 calorie diet.

The larger your frame and the more active your life, the more calories you can consume without storing them. A tiny wisp of a secretary might have to be strict about that 2,000 calorie level, whereas a strapping bricklayer could probably consume 3,000 without gain.

For the average person interested in a typical Longevity Diet day, this could be a typical menu:

Breakfast:	4 ounces Orange Juice
	1 Biscuit Shredded Wheat with milk, one table-spoon honey
	2 Boiled Eggs
	1 cup Coffee, milk, no sugar
Lunch:	1 Tunafish sandwich on whole wheat
	1 portion Cole slaw
	8 ounces Milk
Snack:	1 cup Yogurt
Dinner:	4 ounces Chopped Steak
	1 portion Turnip Greens
	4 ounces Noodles
	2 ounces Cheese
	1 cup Coffe substitute, milk, no sugar
Snack:	1 ounce Cheese

This is a high protein diet, but it is still a balanced diet.

Besides the meat and fish which provide the basic proteins, there is protein in the milk and cheese.

Fat has been added by permitting the whole egg, the yolks being fat. There is also fat in the cheese. Carbohydrates—not the empty kind, but the kind brimming with vitamin and mineral nutrition—are in the fruit juice and vegetables and to a lesser extent in the whole wheat cereal and bread.

The closest to empty calories would be the noodles. If made from whole grain, they are a better food. And if it was rice on the plate, brown rice would be a better food than white rice.

This calorie count is still barely 2,000 calories, leaving a small margin for a dab of margarine (not butter) on the vegetables, some wheat germ over the cereal, or another healthful ingredient you might like to include.

We have kept the balance by increasing portions or quantities, rather than by juggling fats and carbohydrates.

A NON-CALORIC "FOOD" THAT THE BODY NEEDS

The most common cause of death in the United States is coronary heart disease. There is hardly any evidence of this disease in rural Africa.

The most common abdominal operation in the United States is removal of the gall bladder. People who live in rural Africa do not get gallstones.

The most prevalent emergency operation in the United States is appendicitis. There are virtually no cases of inflammation of the appendix in rural Africa.

These three conditions are due to fats and other foods eaten in unbalanced proportions.

But there is one condition Americans get which rural Africans do not get because of what Africans eat and Americans do not eat.

The condition is cancer of the colon.

The reason Africans do not get it: they eat roughage.

Roughage is food that does not stay in the intestinal tract very long. There is nothing in it that the body uses. Because it moves through fast, it takes other waste with it, shortening the time of contact between this waste and the colon.

A technical term for roughage is fiber. The most common roughage food is bran. Bran is the outer-most layer of wheat kernel. Bran is lost when wheat is refined since the bran goes into the industrial garbage. Other foods rich in dietary fiber are the whole grains and many fresh fruits and fresh vegetables.

This roughage is now recognized to help more than just the bowels.

When people eat more high fiber foods in their diet, they excrete more bile acids and fat. Bile acid excretion eliminates internally produced cholesterol, reducing the level of blood cholesterol.

So, roughage in the rural African diet may be the largest contributing factor to their apparent immunity to America's most prevalent diseases.

Americans began to eat less fiber late in the last century when new milling techniques made white flour available. Today, we eat one-fifth of the fiber we ate a century ago.

A slice of whole wheat bread has fewer calories than a slice of white bread. The bran in the wheat and the germ of the wheat add bulk but no calories. Bran is devoid of calories.

Whole bran cereals or part bran cereals are strongly indicated as potentially life extending foods.

Isn't it interesting that nature provides us with vital necessities in practically calorieless ways: fiber, vitamins, minerals.

Coincidentally, the highest calorie foods—the sweets, starches, and fats—are the life-diminishing foods, the non-necessities of life.

Recently, two leading researchers, sponsored by the prestigious World Watch Institute, a non-profit organization devoted to global studies, concluded that the average American's high fat, high calorie diet was responsible for six of the ten leading causes of death. They blamed high fat meats, consumed in large quantities, rich dairy products, refined sugar and refined flour as linked with many forms of cancer and heart disease.

Researchers Erik Eckholm and Frank Record recommended a shift from beef and pork to poultry and fish, lowered consumption of fried foods and butter, cream, and milk. They called for a switch to unsaturated fats, especially substituting margarine for butter, fewer eggs, a decreased consumption of sugar and salt and an increased consumption of whole grains, fresh fruits and vegetables.

In effect, they confirmed the Longevity Diet.

THE MEANING OF A CALORIE

We hear so much about the calorie content of foods that many of us have lost the basic meaning of the calorie.

Actually, a calorie is not a measure of the fattening capability of food. It is a measure of energy. It is defined as the amount of heat required to raise the temperature of one gram of water by 1°C. at normal atmospheric pressure.

Translating calories into pounds, it is commonly accepted that 3,500 excess calories creates one excess pound on the human anatomy.

But the connection between calorie and pound is not iron-clad.

Some foods require more energy to be digested—that is, to have their own energy released—than do others.

Also some foods lower the metabolism, the rate of burning of energy by the body processes, while some foods raise the metabolism and increase this rate of burning.

I have good news for you: meat, poultry and fish take longer to digest, consuming more calories for their own assimilation.

Also, meat, poultry and fish tend to increase the metabolism compared to carbohydrates.

So, you can eat more calories of lean meat, poultry and fish than you can of sweets and starches.

Yes, a calorie is a calorie. But there are variables that take place in the body that make 1,000 calories of one kind of food more fattening than 1,000 calories of another.

Some foods are diuretics or induce perspiration and cause loss of water weight. Others can act as a cathartic and cause more bowel elimination than the weight they supply. We do not get involved with these factors.

But we do enjoy being able to eat protein foods knowing that we are consuming prime nutrition that will supply the least excess calories per ounce of food.

There are two strikes against carbohydrate calories: they usually require fewer calories to digest, yielding a greater net supply. They slow down the furnaces of the body compared to protein, again creating a greater surplus (body fat).

But there are five caloric strikes against fat. Each gram of fat supplies nine calories compared to four for protein and carbohydrate. An equal weight of fat is nearly twice as fattening as anything else.

So, in the calorie league, we are in the right ball park with protein.

HOW THE LONGEVITY DIET AFFECTS
YOUR SEX LIFE

Methuselah lived nine hundred years, according to the Bible. But, according to a popular song based on this fact, what is the use of living if no gal will give in to a man who is nine hundred years.

Well, the lover's lanes of St. Petersburg, Florida, a retirement area, and the sexual competition in homes for the aged have given us new insight into the survival of sexual activity. Senior citizens have their Peyton Place, too; it just does not get gossiped and written about as much.

I have more good news for you.

Longevity on my diet does not yield more years of decrepit existence and senility. Its added years are years of activity, productivity,—and sex.

Sexual activity is directly related to health. Poor eating habits interfere with optimum sexual enjoyment. Hundreds of my clients who have lost significant poundage have volunteered the information that their increased energy levels manifest horizontally as well as vertically. And for every one who is willing to talk about this, there are ten more enjoying similar benefits.

Dr. Elayne Kahn, director of the New York Center for Sexual and Marital Guidance, Inc. and author of "The Whole-Body Health and Sex Book", confirms that many of the "wonder" foods on the Longevity Diet contribute to a better sex life, as do minerals and vitamins.

Iron deficiency causes anemia. Anemic people are poor lovers. Sources of iron include brewer's yeast, wheat germ, turnip greens, spinach, apricots, and molasses. Remember?

Vitamin E deficiency affects the pituitary gland, heart, and bloodstream. You need a normally functioning pituitary and a healthy heart to engage in strenuous sexual activities. Where is Vitamin E found? In wheat germ and vegetable oils (unrefined).

Vitamin A is vital to the reproductive organs. Vitamin B is essenial for the production of sex hormones. Again, this means green vegetables, raw or properly cooked, liver, wheat germ and whole grains.

The same applies to minerals like zinc, potassium, iodine. All are supplied by the "wonder" foods. Zinc is helpful to the male prostate gland, iodine to the thyroid hormones responsible for the sex drive and potassium stimulates female endocrine hormone production.

You will feel good on the Longevity Diet. You will feel younger. You will feel more sexual drive.

HOW TO WORK WONDERS WITH "WONDER" FOODS

Knowing about vitamins and minerals and which are the "wonder" foods is not going to keep you young.

They must become part of your improved way of enjoying food. They must be worked into every day's menu, and into as many recipes and beverages as possible.

High protein foods on the list of "wonder" foods in Chapter 3 are the back-bone of the Longevity Diet. You probably now include these in your daily fare to a degree. They are not new.

However, now the beef must be lean, you should give preference to veal, the leanest of beef. You are also aware of the best parts of poultry and the advantage of fish as a fat-free protein, and you should apply this knowledge.

There are other foods on the "wonder" food list that are not as commonly used, but which I am going to encourage you to use. I am going to do this by bribing you in a way.

At the end of this chapter, you will find a guide that will help you establish a daily calorie limit for yourself.

It is just as important to establish quantity controls on the Longevity Diet as quality controls.

These quantity controls become top priority for overweight persons as the lethal weapon has already hit them, and is hanging on their bodies as human lard.

But even persons with no overweight problem must keep themselves that way. A change of regimen can cause a weight change, so it is good to control quantity through a rough calorie counting process.

The way I am going to bribe you is to call certain "wonder" foods your bonus foods. *They do not have to be counted in your calorie computations.*

Here they are:

- Buttermilk (up to 8 oz.)
- Yogurt (lowfat, unsugared)
- Acidophilus Milk
- Wheat Bran
- Wheat Germ
- Asparagus
- Calorie-less foods
- Sprouts (Alfalfa, Mung Beans, and Others)
- Garlic
- Grapefruit
- Strawberries (fresh)
- Seeds (sesame, Pumpkin, and Sunflower)
- Rose Hips
- Pollen
- Brewer's Yeast (one teaspoon)
- Lecithin and other vitamin and mineral supplements

Do not count these foods within your calorie allotment.

Plump or thin, you may consider the above list my way of toasting your health.

Use one of these foods every meal.

Keep wheat germ on your dining table. Use it for breakfast on cereal and in other ways outlined in Chapter 7.

Keep a dish of sesame or sunflower seeds on a side table as a snack.

Enjoy grapefruit as a dessert. Cook with garlic. Sweeten with pollen. Garnish a salad with sprouts. Keep acidophilus milk fermenting. Favor asparagus or the leafy calorie-free vegetables.

No calorie counting.

But as for the other foods . . .

HOW TO CONTROL PORTIONS FOR LONGER LIFE

Calorie-counting can be fun.

It can also be a bore.

It has always seemed a waste of time to me to see people look up food items and calculate down to the closest calorie when, at best, there can be only ten to twenty percent accuracy.

The food is not uniform. Meat can have more fat or less fat. It can be cooked one way or another. Portions are not weighed out with a scale, just approximated.

So, I say why not just *approximate* calorie counting? You may be a little over here and under there, but it will average out close enough considering other approximations.

Here is a time-saving chart.

ABBREVIATED CALORIE COUNT
OF FOODS CONTAINED IN LONGEVITY DIET

BEEF:	100 calories per ounce.
POULTRY, FISH, VEAL:	60 calories per ounce.
EGG:	75 calories each.
EGG WHITE:	One egg white is 14 calories.
FRUITS:	Will range from 100 calories for 1 medium banana to 18 calories for 1 plum, but a value of 45 calories for 4 ounces of fruit would be considered average.
VEGETABLES:	Green, leafy-type vegetables—35 calories for a four-ounce portion. Other vegetables may range to 80 calories per four-ounce portion.
BREAD:	70 calories per average slice.
RICE, PASTA, NOODLES:	130 calories per four-ounce portion.
CEREAL (Without milk):	80 calories per portion.
MILK (Low fat):	70 calories per eight ounces.
CHEESE:	From low-fat milk—60 calories per ounce. Cheddar, Swiss, etc.—100 calories per ounce. Cottage or similar-low fat—30 calories per ounce.
VEGETABLE JUICE:	55 calories per cup.

FRUIT JUICE: (Unsweetened) 80 calories per cup.

DRY WINE: 45 calories per 3-ounce wine glass.

TEA, COFFEE: 4 calories per 6 ounces.

WATER, PLAIN
SODA WATER: Zero calories.

To determine your weight maintenance calorie intake, you need to take into consideration your present weight, the kind of activities you engage in during the day, and to a lesser degree your age.

The following provides a rule of thumb formula you can use:

FORMULA FOR SETTING LONGEVITY DIET DAILY CALORIC LIMITS

Activity Level	Light	Medium	Heavy
Basic caloric intake	1,400	1,700	2,000
Add this many calories for every pound you weigh over 100	5	10	15
Subtract this many calories for every year your age is over 50	5	7	10

It does not matter whether you are male or female. What matters most is how much you weigh and how active is your day.

Housework with modern conveniences might be rated light; with old-fashioned scrubbing, medium; with gardening thrown in, heavy.

Office work is light. Selling is medium. Most professions, light. Most labor, medium or heavy.

Typical examples: Sarah B. is 62. She is a bookkeeper, weighs 130. Her daily caloric limit would be 1,400 plus 150 (5 x 30) minus 60 (5 x 12) or 1,490.

Joseph V. is a heavy construction worker. He is 40 years old and weighs 170 pounds. His daily caloric limit would be 2,000 plus 1,050 (15 x 70) minus nothing (under 50) or 3,050 calories.

Compute your caloric limit now.

Next, we will talk about beverages, how they affect longevity, and how to drink to your own health.

Chapter 5

Abounding Health on Tap

So far, here is where we stand.

We are beginning to understand how high fat, high sweet, and high starch foods are killers.

We are aware of the benefits of protein, minerals, and vitamins and the wonder foods in which they are to be found.

We are aware of the need for a balanced diet, with 100% or more of our protein foods, at least one wonder food in every meal, and at a total calorie level that keeps us at normal weight.

More about menus later, meanwhile what about liquids?

"Water, water everywhere, but not a drop to drink," bemoaned the ancient mariner. He was surrounded by an ocean of salt water.

Some people feel the same way about fresh water. They see it as "hard," full of inorganic minerals that the body cannot handle and which become deposited on the inside of capillaries and arteries, causing hardening of the arteries and stroke.

These people drink only distilled water—when they can get it. It is available by the bottle at all drugstores and some supermarkets. Drugstores have it because they are compelled by law to use distilled water only in preparing prescriptions. Supermarkets have it because some people are medically required to drink it and thousands more are becoming distilled water conscious.

I see no harm in drinking only distilled water although it can be argued that there are organic minerals, too, in water which the body can utilize. But you will be mineral-rich on the "wonder" foods, so you will not miss the minerals in water.

Nor do I see harm in drinking tap water or well water. If it coats a pan when boiled away, it may be too "hard" and require second thoughts. But generally speaking, municipal water supplies and private wells provide a necessity of life without danger.

Partake generously. It is a natural act. Water is one of the few natural sources of life's necessities that man has not tried to improve on. Except . . .

Except that it may be "spiked" with chlorine, injected with fluorine, and chemicalized in other ways. There are increasing bodies of data that give one pause about the benefits of water so treated. The theory that a little poison is not a dangerous thing collapses in the light of longevity.

Chlorine has been in use since 1908 when it was added to a water supply and found to be effective in combating a typhoid fever epidemic. Today, it is consumed by 100 million Americans.

Recently, researchers have come up with solid evidence that chlorine causes cancer. They have found that the risks of dying from certain types of cancer are more than forty percent greater among chlorinated water drinkers than non-chlorinated.

Dr. Robert Harris, associate director of the toxic chemicals program for the Environmental Defense Fund, a nonprofit consumer interest group, estimates that five to ten percent of all cancer cases are probably caused by chlorination.

Fluorine has been a more recent arrival at the water hole, but has caused more controversy. Chlorine's role of killing bacteria that could cause serious illness can be justified in the light of possible harm to some, but "possible harm to some" looms as a heavy price to pay for fewer dental cavities.

It is just a matter of how conscientious you are about wanting to live longer. You might even be willing to boil your drinking water two or three minutes. It gets rid of the chlorine!

If the high fat, high sugar, or high starch is going to kill you at 75, whereas the cumulative effect of chemicals in the water won't fell you until 85, drink up. But suppose you are shooting for 95?

Remember 95 seems like "old" today, but it may not be tomorrow.

PREPARE NOW FOR A LONGER LIFE WITH WATER

Prestigious scientists are now talking about the possibility of living forever. One day, some say, the DNA code will be unlocked, permitting the synthesizing of living cell matter. One day, others say, man will construct mini-planets in space for five thousand people to live on more cheaply than many suburbanites, where intelligence will expand due to the challenges of space living and where life itself might be extended by the new conditions.

Longevity is approaching. Even if it is not, what have you got to lose by being ready to accept it?

A partly poisoned, partly polluted, partly clogged body is not a good candidate for longevity.

Water, being a daily necessity, passes through our bodies in quantities which can purify or petrify. Some people who live in regions where the water is extremely hard are prone to hardening of the arteries, early senility, and resulting demise.

Be aware of the water you drink, just as you are aware of the food that you eat. What is its source? How has it been treated? What metal conduits or pipes does it pass through before arriving in your home? How does it look? How does it taste? Does it need filtering? Does it need softening?

If in doubt about your drinking water, there are some alternatives. Distilled water is one. There are home distillers that take up little space and convert your tap water into water purer even than raindrops.

Rainwater used to be nature's finest. But today the air is filled with the dust particles and gases of civilization. Raindrops clean the air but in the process become polluted themselves.

Of course, when the rainwater hits the ground, this threat of pollution from factories and sources of effluvia is increasingly present.

Distilled water is safe water if not the best tasting water. You might consider it for use in making coffee, tea or other beverages.

Mineral water is therapeutic, especially as a mild cathartic and occasional restorer of certain rare earth minerals that the body needs in minute quantities but seldom gets. Here again, the usable minerals are mixed with the unusable (inorganic). An occasional drink of mineral water can be beneficial but consult your physician as to specific brands and their appropriateness for you.

COKE, POP, SODA, COLA—THE TRUTH ABOUT SOFT DRINKS

There once was a saying that the sun never set on the British Empire. It is more true now to say that the sun never sets where there is not some Coca Cola, Pepsi Cola, or 7-Up sign in view.

When electricity arrives in some distant area—like it did recently in Bali—the first signs of it are the store refrigerators selling cold soft drinks.

I have just one word to say: Sugar.

About 100 calories of do-nothing-for-you but do-plenty-to-you sugar.

White sugar, at that.

If you drank an eight ounce bottle of soda, you would have to eat several wonder foods that day to make up for the vitamin draining, mineral leaching effects of that 100 calories of sugar. And it would still leave its mark on you in excess calories. Just 100 excess calories a day means ten extra pounds at the end of a year.

William Dufty, a reporter, was suffering from illness after painful illness. Then one day he arranged to meet the ageless film star Gloria Swanson for an interview. Sandwiches and coffee were served and as he reached for the sugar, Miss Swanson said to him, "That stuff is poison. I won't even let it in my house."

Dufty thought about this later and decided to avoid sugar. For the first few days it was like kicking the dope habit. He realized he had become a sugar addict. But then life got better. His illnesses faded. He dropped 65 pounds. His constant fatigue turned into perpetual energy.

Dufty had kept in touch with Gloria Swanson during this

period. They are now married, and he is the author of the best-selling book *Sugar Blues* (Warner).

"Well," you say, "so I'll switch to the diet and low-cal sodas."

I wish I could endorse them. But the substitution may be like jumping out of the fry pan into the fire.

In this case the fire is cancer. The leading sugar substitute is as closely suspected of being as direct a cause of cancer as smoking. This substitute is *saccharin*, the substitute that the United States Food and Drug Administration has been deeply concerned about. On November 15, 1977, the FDA instructed diet soft drink bottlers using saccharin to begin placing cancer warning labels on their products.

The tentative guidelines called for the following warning to be placed on bottles and cartons:

"Use of this product may be hazardous to your health. This product contains saccharin which has been determined to cause cancer in laboratory animals."

Well, are you trapped into drinking water alone? No, there are other choices.

Mrs. Koume Hirakawa, the oldest woman in Japan, died at her home in Osaka, August 8, 1977. She was 108. Her favorite drink was tea.

TEA AND COFFEE
DO NOT SHORTEN LIFE—TRUE OR FALSE?

Tea contains tannic acid. It is said to harden the stomach walls, like leather. Apparently, harder stomach walls do not shorten life as much as other factors. Mrs. Hirakawa's demise was due to lung inflammation—the air she breathed was more dangerous, at least for her, than the liquid she drank, in this case tea.

Coffee contains caffeine. Caffeine is a stimulant. Many health specialists have spoken out against coffee and the damage it can do to the pancreas, nervous system and heart.

Recently, Duke University Medical Center researchers completed a study of the coffee drinking habits of 2,350 adults in rural Evans County, Georgia. They interviewed these people some time ago to see how many cups of coffee a day they drank. Now, nearly five years later, they investigated the cause of 339 deaths that occurred among these people since the interviews.

What they found was that the people who drank as many as five cups of coffee and more were not dying at any greater rate than those who drank little or no coffee.

The researchers did a thorough job of checking on hospital records, autopsy reports, and all other information available on the 339 deaths. According to Dr. Siegfried Heyden, professor of community health sciences at Duke, forty percent of these deaths were due to heart attacks and strokes, in no greater proportion among coffee drinkers.

However, lets take a closer look. Suppose we were to say hypothetically of the fatalites that inorganic salts had been clogging and hardening their capillaries and arteries. Then suppose we were to say this factor had not occurred earlier in their lives. What would eventually kill them? Maybe it would be the coffee.

It is almost like examining the last 339 traffic fatalities and because the victim's coffee habits were the same as the general population, could we say that coffee is not a killer?

We need to keep some reservations about coffee.

If two people were to live perfect lives, totally free of the poisons in food, air, and drink, one drinking only water, and the other drinking only coffee, I would put my chips on the water drinker to outlive the coffee drinker.

But coffee in moderation, in my opinion, must take a back seat to greater threats to our longevity. The three cup drinker is probably in a safer position than the five cup drinker. Naturally, I'm assuming no sugar. Sugar will get you if the coffee does not.

If you tend to be overweight, coffee can aggravate this problem. It is not the calorie content of coffee, it is the caffeine content. As I said before, coffee affects the pancreas. It interferes with its normal function of stabilizing blood sugar content. As a result, coffee causes increases and then decreases in the level of blood sugar. Hence, the feeling of a lift. But the reaction to the lift, the lowering of blood sugar, is often felt as hunger.

Decaffeinated coffee does not cause these blood sugar cycles and false hungers. I would urge overweight people, who will now be in the process of normalizing their weight, to switch to the decaffeinated coffees until weight is normal.

There is caffeine in tea. If overweight, drink weak tea to avoid its hungering effects.

For those who desire to follow in Methuselah's footsteps and avoid even the slightest risks, there are some interesting beverages to consider as substitutes for coffee and tea.

HERB TEAS AND COFFEE SUBSTITUTES

Tea comes from the dried leaves of a shrub called Thea Sinensis. It is found mostly in eastern Asia. The shrub bears white flowers and evergreen leaves. Variations in tea come from the leaves of shrubs in different areas, growing in different soils and at different elevations, also from picking the leaves at different stages of growth and drying or preparing them in different ways.

But it is still tea, and the more standard the brand, the further it is removed from the natural substance through the additions of more processes and additives such as colorants.

The true switch comes not from switching from a standard brand to say green tea, but from switching shrubs.

Health food store shelves are lined with varieties of herb tea too numerous to mention. These, too, are usually made from leaves but also from roots and barks.

Our forefathers learned about what herbs, roots and barks taste good and are beneficial, not only from their own experiments but from the experience of the American Indian.

Each herb tea with a record of long use has a reputation for therapeutic benefits, like alfalfa, said to be valuable in relieving arthritic pain, peppermint said to be soothing to the stomach, and chamomile said to be calming to the nerves and sleep-inducing.

For our purposes, it is probably more important that you investigate these herb teas for the purpose of finding those that taste best to you. The herb teas now being sold include different combinations, so they appeal to many tastes. Some have exotic or descriptive names like the multi-herb: "Red Zinger", "Rose Garden," made of rose hips and hibiscus blossoms; and Magic Mountain's "Sunrise Blend" of chamomile, peppermint and alfalfa.

Besides alfalfa, peppermint, and chamomile, other basic herb teas include comfrey, eucalyptus, foenugreek, ginseng, goldenseal, mandrake, papaya leaves, rose hips, sarsaparilla, sassafras, spearmint, and valerian.

Explore. You may make a beverage discovery.

There are also a few substitutes for coffee. Perhaps the most established of these is Postum, created over 75 years ago. It is made from bran, wheat, and molasses. It is only 12 calories a serving and so almost ignorable from that standpoint. It really needs no sweetening and has a lusty-enough flavor to satisfy most coffee drinkers.

On the other hand, Ovaltine, also around a long time, has more calories—over 100 per serving, largely because it is mixed with milk, not water, and contains sugar.

Some products are being offered as coffee substitutes which are probably a step backward (like pills that purport to give you a lift and are really coffee extract equal to several cups).

Health food stores are likely to carry several coffee substitutes worth trying. An example is the Bragg Coffee Substitute, a blend of California barley, tree-ripened figs, and soy beans. Postum's calories are all carbohydrates. This product is higher in calories, but these calories include a percentage that are protein due to the soy beans.

These days of high coffee prices provide an additional incentive to vary your beverages. In the process you might also feel less nervous and irritable, and able to fall asleep faster. You may also be free of some tars and toxic acids in coffee, and, of course, those pancreatic cycles.

Coffee and tea rate very low on the life threatening list of substitutes we put in our mouths.

The more the Food and Drug Administration looks for cancer-causing agents in our foods and beverages, the more they find. Nitrates and nitrites, as common as the hot dog and bacon, are found to form nitrosamines in the stomach of animals, leading to cancer. They are thought to do the same for humans.

Food colorants and flavorings, like Violet No. 1 and Red Dyes No. 2 and No. 4, are banned by the FDA because they were shown to cause cancer in animals. Other materials like the flavoring used for root beer and vermouth have also been banned.

Pesticides once thought to be harmless to humans, like aldrin, DDT, and dieldrin were found to cause cancer in animals and to leave residues of their poison in foods sold for human consumption.

The list will continue to grow. It now includes saccharin and

once included cyclamates. Regulations will be invoked and re-
voked. All this is man's doing, which is never quite as good as
nature's.

Still, the real dietary villains in Americans are the high fat
foods, the high sugar foods, the high in white flour foods.

Eliminate these fats, sweets and starches, and you take a
giant step in added years.

Eliminate the poisonous additives in our food and beverages
and you take a smaller step in added years.

Eliminate coffee and tea and you take a still smaller step
in the direction of longevity. Of course, eliminating coffee when
you are an excessive drinker is a larger step in the right direction
than if you are a 3-cup a day drinker.

It is up to you to decide whether the small increment—whatever it may be—is worth the loss of the enjoyment you derive from
the traditional brews.

ALCOHOL—A MINUS OR PLUS?

Excessive alcohol consumption is definitely a killer.

Still, moderate amounts of wine have been shown to be good
for the heart.

In order to place each of these statements into proper longevity perspective, let's examine them more closely.

Excessive drinking is a well-known killer. Some softhearted
sots drink themselves under the table because they think it's the
thing to do. The next they know, their habit is out of control and
they have drunk themselves under six feet of dirt.

Other excessive drinkers become more and more dependent
on alcohol until it's too late. Too late means usually cancer or
cirrhosis of the liver. The liver actually "lives" you; its functions
are so diverse and so vital. No liver, no you.

Doctors now realize the unborn child can be adversely affected by a drinking mother. The National Institute on Alcohol
Abuse and Alcoholism has warned that women who take more
than two drinks a day during pregnancy run the risk of giving birth
to physically deformed and mentally retarded babies.

Excessive drinking also leads to cancer of the esophagus,
mouth, larynx and throat, without mentioning such side effects
as traffic death.

Moderate amounts of wine might be good for you.

"Wine," said Euripides, "removes the cares pressing on the minds of sorrowing souls."

But wine has a much broader role in human life. The Hebrews called wine, "The foremost of medicines." St. Paul counseled, "Drink no longer water, but use a little wine for thy stomach's sake and thine infirmities."

Today, wine is occasionally used as a tranquilizer. It is certainly safer than most. Wine has also been prescribed for ulcer therapy. Diabetic patients are permitted to indulge in table wines that contain little or no grape sugar. There is a growing belief that wine is good therapy for older people in hospitals and nursing homes.

Wine is pretty close to being as much food as it is beverage. It contains carbohydrates, several vitamins, and a dozen or more minerals. But it might be as much good medicine as it is food.

Research at the U. S. National Institutes of Health, reported in the journal of the British Medical Association, showed that men who drink about 12 glasses of wine a week have proportions of different kinds of fat in their bloodstreams which differ from those of teetotalers. The difference means a lower risk of coronary thrombosis.

The same is true of equivalent amounts of beer or hard liquor, so it is apparently the alcohol—in one or two shots a day—that corrects the bloodstream fat.

So here we have another case of a little being benign, and a lot being lethal.

Overweight people are in double jeopardy. They stand to gain weight as they damage their livers.

Some tips to drinkers who must watch their weight:

- Favor dry wine over sweet wine.
- Beer is a weighty problem,—125 calories per 8 oz. glass. Even if you cut your food calories to accommodate beer, you shortchange yourself on nutrition.
- Straight shots of hard liquor are to be preferred over cocktails or mixes which are likely to have sugar.
- Avoid cordials,—1 oz. can have almost as many calories as 8 oz. of beer.

Well, so much for stimulants. What does that leave us?

THE BEST WAYS TO QUENCH THIRST

Coffee, tea, dry wine and hard liquor (straight) might be considered to be social drinks. In moderation, they provide solutions rather than cause problems.

There are substitutes for coffee and tea which do not have to be moderated. Some are delicious cold as well as hot.

Water is your best thirst quencher, soft drinks your worst. But there are still a world of thirst quenchers open to you.

The fruit juices and vegetable juices, especially those mentioned under the "wonder" foods are excellent thirst quenchers. However, you need to count about 100 calories for each 5 ounce glass of fruit juice. Vegetable juice has about half as many calories.

Robert A., a counselor and health-minded, was gaining weight for the first time in his life. Even in his fifties he had not succumbed to paunchiness. Now at 60, he did not welcome such a problem, yet the scale would not go away. On examination of his eating habits, we found that Robert had acquired a new drink—apple juice.

"It is excellent for digestion," he insisted, "Remember, too, an apple a day . . ."

The way Robert was hitting that apple juice, the doctor would not be kept away very long. I convinced him an apple eaten, with the additional minerals, vitamins and roughage of the pulp and skin, was a better bet.

He switched to tomato juice and his weight returned to normal.

Vegetable juices are to be preferred over fruit juices as thirst quenchers, just on a calorie for calorie comparison; grapefruit juice is a good thirst quencher and quite low in calories compared to the other fruit juices. Apple, orange, and grape are comparatively high in calories.

One way to get more thirst quenching pleasure per calorie of juice is to add ice and some water, especially if you prefer iced drinks. There is plenty of flavor in natural juice, and even with 50 percent water, it holds up well in taste.

Continuing down the list of available thirst quenchers we find:

- Mineral water
- Club soda
- Buttermilk
- Skim milk
- Non-fat dry milk

Mineral water is a "wonder" food thanks to its minerals. It has no calories. You may or may not like its taste. Still it quenches and cleanses.

Club soda is carbonated water. It sparkles and tingles. It has no sugar. It is not better than water, but it is better than its sugared cousins.

Regular milk is becoming controversial as an adult beverage. I don't want to enter the controversy because there is little scientific evidence yet one way or the other. Even mother's milk is coming under fire. DDT, dieldrin, and other chemicals considered to be dangerous have been found in the breast milk of hundreds of women tested. Still, mother's milk is baby's best bet.

Buttermilk is low in calories and has a thirst quenching zing to it. Also, it is found in the life styles of long-lived people. Skim milk is regular milk with the animal fat removed. It is more watery and thirst quenching than regular milk and contains more protein.

Powdered milk (not evaporated or condensed) is a safe milk substitute, thirst quenching and low in calories.

PETRIE'S NATURAL PROTEIN LONGEVITY DRINKS

If you are willing to nourish your body with "wonder" foods while you quench your thirst, I invite you into my kitchen. I have a few personal favorites that I would like to share with you.

Here is a drink that is a complete satisfying breakfast:

PETRIE'S PROTEIN "BREAKFAST IN A GLASS"

3/4 C. Acidolphilus milk or Yogurt thinned with milk
1 ripe banana
2 t. Tahini (sesame seed butter)
2 t. sunflower meal
½ t. Brewers Yeast

2 t. wheat germ
2 T. natural honey
1 t. Vanilla
2 t. soy flour
1 t. Calcium Lactate powder
Generous dash of nutmeg and cinnamon

Blend all together in blender. Serve at once. For one.

Here is my special blend of spices for hot tea:

PETRIE'S SPICE OF LIFE TEA

Boil 2½ C. water
Add 8 whole cardomom seeds
6   whole cloves
12 whole peppercorns
2   thin slices fresh ginger (or ½ t. dried ginger)
½ cinnamon stick

Boil altogether for 25 minutes. Lemon to taste. Serves two.

Here is another healthful hot drink:

PETRIE'S HOT PROTEIN PUNCH

1 C. milk (skim or reconstituted dry milk)
1½ T. honey
1 T. ground blanched almonds
1 T. sunflower meal
1/8 t. nutmeg, cinnamon
1 cardamon seed crushed (optional)

Bring milk almost to a boil. Lower heat to simmer and add honey and spices. Stir well and cook five minutes. Serves one.

Now, you are probably just as good an improvisor as I am. So I don't represent these drinks to be the most delicious or even the most life-prolonging. I happen to like them and I find there is more fun to concocting these kinds of drinks at a kitchen counter than mixing drinks behind a bar.

There is one drink I make which really makes the body cells come to attention.

It combines three powerful longevity foods into one fairly

low calorie and high vitality drink. Try it. Make it part of an occasional day's menu.

Two favorite foods of the incredible Soviet Abkhasians are yogurt and buttermilk. Both contain predigested protein that is instantly available to your body for repairing old cells and building new ones. Both contain lactic acid to sweep your cells clean of metabolic debris and infuse them with new life.

What yogurt and buttermilk are to the long-lived Soviet Abkhasians, apricots are to the fabled Pakastani Hunzas. Apricots contain an abundance of strength-promoting iron, anti-infective, anti-aging vitamin A and perhaps a certain secret something that prompts the Hunzas to claim the apricot their prime longevity-promoting food.

PETRIE'S NATURAL PROTEIN LONGEVITY DRINK
(Makes three 6 oz. servings—each serving 93 calories)

Mix in blender 1 cup plain skim milk yogurt,
1 cup buttermilk
3½ - 4 oz. of fresh or canned unsweetened aprocots (approximately
4 to 5 apricots)
Mix and serve as a healthful substitution for any meal or take as a mid-morning or afternoon snack . . .

To your health!

Chapter 6

Cooking for a Longer Life

The Croatians are a long-lived people. They attribute their extra years to drinking slivovitz, a plum brandy.

But they have nobody in Croatia like our Charlie Smith. A former slave, Charlie Smith is 135 as this is being written in late 1977. Smith's age has been confirmed by Social Security records. It came to light when he was found to be picking citrus fruit near Lakeland, Florida in 1957 at the age of 115.

Slivovitz? Florida citrus? What is the real fountain of youth?

There are a number of theories on why aging occurs. To name just a few:

- *Stress Theory.* The more stress the greater and faster the breakdown. Stress includes poor nutrition, temperature extremes, and disease.
- *Fast Metabolism Theory.* The greater the rate of metabolism, due largely to excessive eating, the shorter the life span.
- *Waste Product Theory.* The accumulation of the waste products of metabolism interfere with natural functions of vital systems.
- *Free Radical Theory.* Pieces, called free radicals, break off

from chemical compounds in the body and combine with
other materials to cause aging.

- *Oxidation Theory*. Like rust, when oxygen enters a molecule, it changes its nature causing aging.
- *Protein Synthesis Theory*. Nucleic acids are mismatched
as communications breakdown between DNA and RNA.
- *Cross-Linkage Theory*. Molecules in tissues begin to inter-
connect, reducing the efficiency of their functioning.

There are more. But these seem to be the ones most seriously
regarded today. I have placed them in this order to point out the
importance of nutrients in all,—most obvious in the first, perhaps
least obvious in the last.

The stress theory includes poor nutrition as a major factor of
stress. The fast metabolism deplores overeating. The waste product
theory points the finger, at least partially, at food additives. The
free radical theory and oxidation theories point to the efficacy of
Vitamin E which helps neutralize free radicals and acts as an anti-
oxidant. The protein synthesis theory indicates the advantage of
complete proteins in the diet. Perhaps only the cross-linkage
theory does not have an obvious link with nutrition, but with six
out of seven pointing to nutrition, it is a good bet that this is the
correct direction to go, even should the seventh theory prove
valid.

Little wonder that Ross and Bras, after their research with
animals, reported emphatically that "What we have done here is
to confirm the fact that under natural conditions, there is a relationship between dietary habits and life span."

The Longevity Diet touches all of the bases identified by
present scientific theories.

So far, we have spotlighted the "wonder" foods that contain
what the body needs for maximum nutrition, especially the protein, minerals and vitamins.

We have pointed the finger at the enemies to longevity, too,
naming fats and the empty calories of white sugar and white flour
as the most insidious.

We have rung the obesity alarm, and pointed out the danger
of every excess pound.

We have looked at the major contaminants in food and drink

and detailed the major mistakes we make in selecting daily beverages.

Yet, you can pick all the right foods and all the right beverages and still lose years off your life nutritionally. You can do all the right things in the supermarkets and health food stores, then do all the wrong things in your kitchen and be back where you started from.

In this chapter we will address ourselves to avoiding the pitfalls in food preparation that negate nutrition. We will stress cooking for maximum good taste and longevity.

In the next chapter we will help you to create interesting meals with infinite diversity to make every healthful eating day more exciting than the last. And in the chapter that follows that, we will provide scores of recipes using "wonder" foods.

Shall we proceed to the kitchen?

HOW COOKING CAN MAKE OR BREAK NUTRIENTS

Mrs. Charlotte L. got cold after cold. Her friends pointed to two causes: (1) She had marital problems; (2) She was not getting enough Vitamin C.

There they were—the mental cause and the physical cause. It had to be one or the other or both.

Charlotte solved her marital problems, and also made Vitamain C vegetables and fruits a daily habit.

Yet, she still got colds. Now what? That was the question she put to me. I started questioning her kitchen habits. Exposure to air destroys certain vitamins. So do other factors. I went down the list. Then it struck me.

"What kind of pots do you cook in?"

"Copper," Charlotte replied.

"That's it," I exclaimed, feeling a bit like Sherlock Holmes, "copper destroys vitamin C on contact."

How you store your foods, the pots you use to prepare them, and the materials of preparation are just as important as starting with the right foods. Improper storage, handling and cooking can convert fresh nutritious food into food as dead as white bread.

Copper is excellent cookware. It conducts heat quickly and evenly from the range to all parts of the pot or pan, minimizing scorching at the center and poorly cooked food at the sides. But it must be lined copper.

Usually, copperware is lined with stainless steel. Steel is a relatively benign metal and does not chemically affect food nutrients. The stainless steel is metallurgically "married" to the inside of copper pots and pans these days, so that it lasts the lifetime of the pot. Should copper show through on your cooking surface, the best thing you can do is hang that particular pot or pan on the wall as decoration.

There is a way to get these pots relined. It is called "tinning." It is also a protector against copper.

Methods of cooking also affect the nutrient content. Generally speaking, contact with high heat can destroy many minerals, and cooking water can dissolve many vitamins.

Consequently, there are two basic principles to follow:

1. Give preference to baking, roasting, and broiling over frying.
2. Use a minimum of cooking water, just enough to prevent scorching, and use the residue of such cooking water for soups and sauces.

Frying that involves deep fat is doubly undesirable. You kill the nutrients you want and inject what you do not want—fat. There are a number of pan sprays that permit fat-less frying. This is a step to the good. There are also heavy griddles which, once greased, can be used over and over if cleaned by wiping.

Since the degree of heat is the critical factor, sauteeing over medium heat for a longer time is better than quick intense heat.

The Chinese wok that lifts the food over the burner is a healthier utensil to use than the frying pan for that same reason.

Cooking vegetables by "stir fry" is a favorite Chinese method. The surface of the wok is not as hot as direct contact pans. The vegetables are cut into small pieces, the wok is oiled, and the food is stirred, scooped and turned in the heated wok for just a minute or two. The food retains its color, flavor and nutrients. Sometimes, a little broth is added and the vegetables are permitted to simmer to become tender but still crisp.

Another similar technique is now used in the West: A stainless steel basket can be placed in an ordinary pot to keep the vegetables free of cooking water. The resulting steaming process seals in all the nutrients and flavor.

FAT-FREE COOKING IS TOP PRIORITY

I watched Jack A. eat his steak. He had just finished telling me how he avoids fried foods of all types. He loves chicken but will drive a mile to pick up the roasted or "broasted" rather than the more popular and readily available fried chicken.

It was a broiled sirloin steak. "Medium rare," he had told the waiter. Now he was enjoying it—fat and all.

Jack was not a client so I offered him no uninvited advice, but can you guess what I would have told him?

Yes, Jack made his first mistake when he ordered his steak medium rare. Heat does not harm meat. In fact, heat helps to make meat leaner. It melts away fat. Jack's medium rare steak had just as much if not more fat in it than the fried chicken he knew not to eat.

And, of course, Jack should have trimmed the fat from every mouthful and eaten just the meat. Just as bacon tastes good, the fat on beef tastes good with the meat. But the price in health can be prohibitive.

In 1976 Americans consumed a record amount of "visible" fat. According to the U. S. Department of Agriculture, the average per person was 56 pounds. USDA officials predicted this would rise to 60 pounds by 1985. "Visible" fats are butter, margarine, shortenings, and salad dressings. It does not even include the fat visible on meats, much less the fat within the flesh of meat, and in cheese, milk, eggs and other foods.

We need to recognize fats, visible or not, and do something about them. One place is in the supermarket. We can minimize fatty products on our shopping lists. Another place to be careful is the kitchen. We can cook with as little oil and fat as possible. The third place to watch is the table. Are you listening, Jack?

STORING FOODS
FOR MINIMUM LOSS OF NUTRIENTS

The more nutritious a food, the more important it is to mold, insects, rodents, and scavengers.

You can keep white bread around for quite a while. It will get stale before it will get anything else. Ants, cockroaches and other bugs turn their noses up at it. Even fungi seek more fertile ground to grow.

Whole wheat flour must be kept refrigerated or it will succumb to nature's living organisms that know a good thing. Many other foods obtained at a health food store need to be refrigerated despite your never having had to refrigerate their purified, refined, and preserved supermarket cousins.

Our omnipresent eroder of the nutrition in food is oxygen.

Fruits and vegetables survive better than do meats and poultry. But once peeled or sliced, even fruits and vegetables loss their goodness quickly. Stored as nature grew them, they will keep their goodness for days, but also they will continue to ripen and can reach the point of over-ripeness or rotten practically overnight. Here, too, refrigeration slows the process.

Ideally, local produce should be eaten instead of produce that has had to be harvested or picked unripe in order to better last out a long trip. Then, when purchased, it should be eaten as soon as possible. Even with today's refrigeration facilities, every day saps nutrition from fresh fruit and fresh vegetables.

That is why the canning, bottling and freezing process have proved economically valuable. And that is why preservatives such as sugar and chemicals are added. Shelf life of the product is improved. But your life will not be improved.

Even canned and bottled goods, taken for granted by purveyors as able to last indefinitely in terms of days, weeks, and months, are waking up to some rude realities. Baby food spoils quite fast, even sealed in jars. All cans and jars need to be dated, lest first in, first out handling methods create overly stored inventory.

Frozen fruits and vegetables are not immune from spoilage, albeit at an extremely slow rate. How does the package look? Is it damaged, beat up, torn? Pick a newer looking one.

You will be buying fresh produce more than frozen. Frozen produce is often precooked and you have no control over how much this cooking has robbed the food of its heat sensitive minerals and water soluble vitamins.

Sugar is going to be in practically all prepared foods these days, even frozen. Would you believe that food processors are putting sugar into salami and bologna, even hot dogs?

A check of labels will show you that there is sugar in canned peas, canned corn, and canned tomatoes. There is sugar in Gerber's Sweiback toast, in Breyer's "all natural yogurt" and "Quaker 100% Natural Cereal."

Yes, sugar is even injected into prepared "health" foods.

Decide to *store* fresh ingredients yourself and do your own *preparation.* Why put your life in other's hands?

Here are some pointers:

1. Do not peel fruits or vegetables until ready to cook or use.
2. Do not grind, chop, or cut meat until ready to cook.
3. Do not blend juices until ready to drink.
4. Refrigerate natural grains to slow their spoilage, even though in unopened bags.
5. Store leftovers in glass, plastic or ceramic containers, preferably with airtight covers or plastic wrap.
6. Refrigerate or freeze leftovers.
7. Count on your refrigerator to store foods for not more than a week, your freezer for no more than a month.

COMMON INGREDIENTS
THAT CAUSE COMMON AILMENTS

Food properly bought and properly stored is ready for proper preparation.

If I were to take a look into your kitchen, I would see a number of ingredients used in food preparation that are common to kitchens everywhere.

Yes, there are the salt and the pepper. And there are the ketchup and mayonnaise.

If you are going to buy "wonder" foods and then use these seasonings and spreads, the wonder will be that you reach your full life expectancy.

Let's talk about salt.

Salt comes under attack from the medical profession when high blood pressure occurs, and occasionally when there are allergic reactions. The fact is that Americans consume ten times the amount of salt they really need, according to Dr. Jean Mayer of Harvard.

"Salt to taste" is seen on recipes. Actually our taste buds have been seduced by salt as surely as they have been by sugar.

Table salt is about 60 percent chlorine and 40 percent sodium. When the chlorine is released, it helps to make hydrochloric acid used by the stomach to digest protein. The sodium that is released goes into the bloodstream where its presence, in balanced quantities, is vital.

Getting enough salt has been almost as important in man's early political history as getting enough water. Many a tribal battle was fought over salt.

Today's distribution systems supply most people with an abundance of salt, even though the physical need for salt has been eclipsed by the sensory need. People have become addicted to the taste of salt.

Today, food processors put salt into just about everything. Canned soup is salted. Canned vegetables contain salt. Processed meats have lots of salt added. So does cheese, bread, even fish from the already salty sea. Even water that has been softened has salt in it.

Then these products are heated or otherwise prepared in the kitchen with a pinch of more salt added. Then at the table you hear, "Pass the salt."

What is all that salt doing to the body?

To find the answer to this question, scientists compared peoples that were living with salt and without. F. W. Lowenstein looked at the health of two tribes adjacent to each other in the Brazil jungle. The Mundurueus tribe had been introduced to salt and used it abundantly. The people lived quite primitively yet their blood pressure tended to rise as they got older.

The other tribes, the Carajos, had no contact with civilization and used no salt. They had no hypertension at all. Older people had the same blood pressure as younger people.

Other studies found the same results in Malaysia, New Guinea, the Solomon Islands, and Uganda. No salt, no hypertension.

We get all the natural organic salt we need, easily assimilated by the body, in vegetables, meat and eggs. If you add it to food in the kitchen, you could be adding trouble.

Of course, if you have super kidneys, large arteries and a strong heart, something else will be your weak link in the chain of life. But why bet against yourself?

"How about in hot weather" you ask. Yes, the body needs more salt in hot weather, but it is probably already getting more salt than it needs.

The late Paul Bragg, even in his vigorous nineties, would tell the story about his World War I days when he never took the salt tablets provided by the army and still had more energy than the others. Later, in an attempt to prove his point, he challenged an army squad to hike with him through the heat of Death Valley with their salt tablets. Every one succumbed to nausea or heat prostration, except Bragg.

If a low salt diet can relieve hypertension, allergy, migraine, dizziness and many other ailments, why not avoid excess salt and prevent these problems.

A quarter ounce less salt a day can equal a full ounce of prevention.

HOW TO BRING OUT THE FULL FLAVOR OF FOOD WITHOUT USING SALT

Herb teas afford a healthful hot brew, free of caffeine. In the same way, herbs help man flavor his meats and casseroles in ways that far exceed the advantages of salt, without its disadvantages.

If you must keep some salt in the kitchen, keep iodized salt or a salt substitute like kelp, a type of seaweed ground into powder and available at health food stores.

But begin to use herbs in cooking. Stand in front of the herb shelves at the supermarket and research for rosemary, oregano, dill, paprika and bay leaves. Try the oregano on eggs. Try rosemary and paprika in your stews. Put a bay leaf in the roasting pan.

Spices are no jeopardy to health when used in moderation. But lots of pepper, chile and hot pepper sauces are known to cause vasodilation in some people—an expansion of the blood vessels.

This appears on the face as a blushing condition similarly to the flushed face that broken capillaries produce for an alcoholic.

I know of no other warning to issue for other kinds of spices, but perhaps the rule that is always best to follow is indeed: moderation.

Here are a few herbs and spices and some of their recommended uses to bring out the full flavor of "wonder" foods and to break the salt addiction:

Allspice:	Add several whole allspice to the water when boiling shrimp or poaching fish. Also good in stews, roasts, soups, and in fricasseeing chicken.
Anise Seed:	Sprinkle on bland cheese to enhance flavor. Dip raw fruit into the seed for an off-beat flavor.
Basil leaves:	Try it on scrambled eggs and in fish chowders and stews. Add it when cooking tomato dishes.
Bay leaf:	Try in tomato juice. Put two or three bay leaves in the lamb or veal roasting pan. A must when you make tomato sauce.
Celery seed:	Good to put into meat loaf to help replace bread. Try it in cabbage and other cooked vegetables.
Cloves:	Popular for adding to cider for a hot drink. Add to cooking water when preparing squash, carrots or beets, then remove.
Dill seed:	Sprinkle lamb chops with dill seeds before broiling, or add to the lamb stew. Use it with cucumber and in tossed green salads.
Fennel seed:	Good on mild cheeses, seafood, and rice.
Ginger root:	Add the root or its powdered equivalent to stews or soup. A must when cooking meat Oriental-style.

Marjoram:	You'll recognize this taste. Used by experts in meatballs and rubbed on chicken before cooking. Often added to salads.
Nutmeg:	Can create a fancy dessert out of simple puddings and fruit desserts.
Oregano leaves:	Add to vegetable juices for taste. Also a taste booster for tomato sauce.
Rosemary leaves:	Try in fruit punch, but also versatile for soups and stews. Add a pinch to omelets and fish.
Saffron:	Turns a fish stew into Bouillabaisse. A little added to rice makes a rice pilaff taste special.
Tarragon:	Rub on fish before broiling or baking. Use in salad dressing. Also versatile for meats, eggs, etc.
Thyme:	Use it in vegetable juices, also clam juice and broth. Adds flavor to most vegetables.

THE POISONS IN OUR KITCHEN

White sugar, white flour, white salt,—all detrimental to our health and shorteners of life.

What is the color of sodium silicoaluminate? Or dipotassium phosphate? Is carboxymethyl cellulose also white, or sodium caseinate?

These happen to be some of the ingredients besides salt and sugar in instant cocoa preparations. The late nutritionist Adele Davis used to say, "If you cannot pronounce it, don't eat it."

"But they're great for making a chocolate sauce," protested a neighbor of mine, "and they save you so much time."

"Chemicals cost you time," I replied. "You lose more time off your life than you save at the kitchen counter."

Most ketchups are relatively free of chemicals but they do contain sugar.

Mayonnaise is relatively free of chemicals but it does have

egg yolk—animal fat. And how can you be sure the oil used is not rancid?

You might try to make your own ketchup without sugar by blending tomato paste with some of the herbs and spices described earlier in this chapter.

You might try to make your own mayonnaise. Here is a recipe:

> 2 eggs
> 1/8 teaspoon white pepper
> 1/2 teaspoon dry mustard
> 1/8 teaspoon paprika
> 2 tablespoons lemon juice
> 1 cup olive oil or sesame oil
>
> *Make sure all ingredients are at room temperature. Put all the ingredients except the oil in a blender, cover and blend at medium speed for a few seconds. Gradually add oil and continue blending until all oil has been added and thoroughly mixed. Store in refrigerator.*

You can make a mayonnaise substitute free of animal fat with tahini which is sesame paste. Just add lemon juice, water and seasoning, and blend.

If you make it yourself—sauce, dressing, stuffing, gravy, spread—you know what it is in it.

If it is processed to save your time, it will contain chemicals that may not be recognized as dangerous but which right now are taking years off lives.

It takes time before the detrimental effects of some of these food additives become known. Colorants that have been used for years are now suspected of being cancer-causing.

Take the "pill." No, maybe you better not. A continuing study in Great Britain has revised upwards its original estimate of the death rate associated with the oral contraceptive taken by women. Originally, only blood clots, strokes, and heart attacks were considered to be pill-connected. Now it is found that a wider range of circulatory diseases, heart diseases, hemorrhages, and high blood pressure are closely associated with "the pill."

Most medicines have their contra-indications, but because of their aid to the particular health crisis, the slight risk can validly be taken.

But what validates the risk of putting monosodium glutamate on your food? This is the product known in the Orient as Ajinomoto and here as Accent. Even if you are not susceptible to the so-called Chinese restaurant syndrome where this "gourmet powder" is used—the dizziness, headache, etc.—you may be storing up unwanted conditions for the future.

Dr. Girard W. Campbell of Long Island, N.Y.* has been relieving arthritis patients of their crippling pains largely by diet. Part of that diet includes avoiding all processed foods. He points the finger of accusation especially at monosodium glutamate and such other tongue twisters as disodium dihydrogen phosphatase, sorbitan-monostearate, and di-potassium phosphate.

His accusation of sodium nitrate and sodium nitrate used in prepared meats like hot dogs is now receiving some confirmation from other sources. Other common additives he "fingers" are the so-called U. S. certified food colors, sulphur dioxide used for drying fruits, and benzoate of soda.

THE MEANING TO YOU
OF "NATURAL" INGREDIENTS

Which box of eggs would you rather buy, Box A or Box B?

Box A comes from a farm where chickens roam and peck. They roost in comfortable quarters, sleep at night, lay eggs in the daytime.

Box B comes from a poultry establishment where the chickens hardly see the light of day. They are cooped up in wire cages, unable to run about and peck. They are given prepared, perhaps even processed, feed. The lights are kept on at night so they will lay eggs 24 hours a day.

Of course, you would rather have Box A. Were you to cook Box A eggs alongside of Box B eggs, the Box A eggs would exhibit a thick white that stands up well around a full-colored firm yoke compared to Box B eggs. The taste of Box A eggs would be more delicate and mellow compared to the others.

Well, I have some bad news for you. That choice does not exist for most urban Americans. Naturally, produced eggs are not as economically rewarding to the farmer or producer.

Even farmers who believe in the organic or natural egg and

who see the need for chickens to live and scratch naturally are figuring out unnatural ways to mass produce, imitating nature. They provide wire mesh floors as the commercial growers but add a scratching area lined with corn cobs. They make many improvements over the other mass producers in their effort to mass produce natural eggs, but you cannot improve on our nature.

Soon Box A will disappear completely and the closest to a natural organic egg in urban markets will be the nearly natural egg.

This has been the problem throughout the so-called health food industry. How do you make it pay? To eke out that margin of profit, you have to mass produce and lower costs. You also have to extend shelf life to minimize spoilage.

Yogurt is now fraternizing with some strange bedfellows. You are better off making your own yogurt from yogurt starters at health food stores. Take a typical frozen yogurt. The top of the carton in my hand as I write describes the contents: "Cultured low fat milk, non-fat milk solids." So far so good.

"Sugar, cream, corn syrup solids." Bulgaria was never like this.

And then there is "sodium nitrate, mono and diglycerides, citric acid, polysorbate 80, artificial flavor and artificial coloring."

End of case.

Maybe the entire health food industry will one day succumb to economic competition. The customers may live to see that day, but the non-customers may not.

Add years to your life by betting on nature's ways as superior to man's ways. Nature built your body. It was not designed in a drafting room, manufactured in a factory, and put together in an assembly plant. Man has not come close to being able to produce this magnificent organism.

Nature knows best.

Avoid man-made products or man-tampered-with products wherever possible. Choose nature, the taste is better, the nutrition is better.

In some cases these differences may appear small. "Why go to

---

*"The Doctor's Proven New Home Cure for Arthritis," Parker Publishing Co., 1972.

a lot of trouble for a tiny advantage," you say. "Anyway something else will probably get me in the end."

Maybe you are right. But the Longevity Diet to be most effective must not compromise. Favor the natural. Make your own instead of buying ready-made.

And look both ways before crossing the street.

THE TEN KITCHEN COMMANDMENTS
FOR LONGEVITY

In talking about the preference of natural over processed, we can begin to cloud the issue.

The goal is to live longer. The main threats to our longer life are too much fat and empty carbohydrates at the expense of protein.

If you can handle this threat, you are getting the most of the Longevity Diet benefit in added years. I could say all the rest of the dietary steps mentioned are just icing on the cake, but I won't.

In order to keep this major thrust in proper perspective, let me list the steps you need to take in their order of priority to create the proper "atmosphere" in your kitchen for longevity meals.

1. Have enough lean meat, fish, and poultry to maintain high protein menus.

2. Avoid the use of fats in cooking as much as possible. Limit the use of butter, and if you have a weight problem, of margarine and oils.

3. Cook and prepare without sugar and flour. Do not use recipes that require sugar or bread crumbs, sweetening or dough.

4. Stock your kitchen with as many "wonder" foods as possible. Aim for eating only "wonder" foods; be happy with no less than two or three every meal, one as an absolute minimum.

5. Keep a supply of mineral and vitamin supplements on hand. Make them a daily habit. Be especially interested in the B complex, C and E.

6. Use a vegetable substitute for ordinary salt, or re-educate your taste buds to appreciate the unsalted, natural taste of food.

7. Buy fresh fruit and produce when possible. Favor local produce where available. Prefer frozen to canned or bottled.

8. Cook in ways to preserve natural goodness—avoid high temperatures and use minimum water.

9. Avoid products that are preserved, homogenized, colored, and in other ways chemically treated. Read the labels. The bigger the words, the bigger the risk.

10. Look for organic and natural products; this means natural farming methods that do not use chemical sprays and fertilizers that leave their mark on the product and in you.

You might call these your ten commandments for maintaining a longevity kitchen, providing the best nutrition that planet earth can provide you and your family.

In the next chapter, I will help you put together recipes that observe these ten principles.

Chapter 7

Longevity Recipes
Using "Wonder Foods"

In this chapter you will find new ways to use the "wonder" foods described in Chapter 3.

The recipes given are not original. They have been acquired over the years, perhaps adapted, improved, changed, and shared with my clients and friends alike.

They are aimed at utilizing high protein ingredients, preferably plant protein. Their thrust is to low fat, preferably polyunsaturated. They stear clear as much as possible of sugar, salt, and white flour. They call for methods of cooking which, wherever possible, avoid frying or the use of high heat that might destroy some nutritional values. They use minimal cooking water which, when thrown down the sink, takes valuable vitamins with it.

There is no requirement to use these recipes. They are here to stimulate your own creative ideas on how to use more of the "wonder" foods with more frequency in your every day fare.

Try every "wonder" food. The more you try, the more "wonder" foods you will discover you greatly enjoy. Be adventurous, adaptive, open-minded. Only through such an expanded consciousness can you break out of the sugar-flour trance that your taste buds have been hypnotized into by "civilized" foods.

In all of these recipes: T = tablespoon
t = teaspoon
C = cup

BEEF—LEAN CUTS

Flank Steak
(for 2)

1 lb. flank steak
1 clove garlic
1 T soy sauce
½ t honey
1½ T sherry

Remove all fat. Rub garlic on both sides. Combine next three ingredients. Smear on the steak and let stand several hours. Broil only a few minutes on each side. Slice on an angle and serve.

EGG WHITES

The classic recipe for egg-whites is a confection known as merangue shells. However, sugar must be used. We prefer to use egg-whites in recipes such as the following:

Fruit Foam

1 egg-white
1 T honey
1½ C grapefruit juice, chilled

Beat egg white till stiff. Beat in the honey. Add the juice and pour into glasses garnished with mint leaves.

FISH AND SARDINES

Chinese Steamed Fish

3 lb. fish, such as sea bass or snapper
1 clove garlic, crushed
½ to 1 t grated ginger root
2 minced scallions
1½ T fermented black bean paste (available in Oriental stores)
3 T fine soy sauce
1 T sherry
½ T honey
1 T sesame or peanut oil

Have whole fish scaled and cleaned. Leave on head or tail. Score on both sides. Combine bean paste and garlic and mix together with rest of ingredients. Spread over fish. Steam until flesh is transparent—about 20 minutes. You can make a steamer out of a broiling pan. Fill with about ½ inch of water. Place fish on a rack. Cover with heavy-duty aluminum.

Sardines and Cabbage

3 C shredded cabbage (Chinese or regular)
1 can sardines with oil
1 t lemon juice
pepper

Place cabbage on platter. Drizzle with half of the lemon juice, sprinkle with freshly ground pepper and lightly toss. Carefully arrange sardines on bed of cabbage. Pour rest of lemon juice over them. Serve with brown rice.

CHICKEN

Almond Chicken Salad
(For 2)

1 C sliced cooked chicken breast
1/3 C almonds or cashews, chopped
1 chopped pimento or sweet pepper
1 C diced celery
1 t chopped green onions

Mix with home-made mayonnaise and serve in papaya shells or on salad greens.

Chicken Curry
(For 2)

4 chicken pieces, skinned
1 small onion, minced
¼ C oil
1 clove garlic, minced
Curry powder to taste
½ C yogurt
½ T paprika
dash of dried ginger
1 small tomato, chopped

Saute onions and garlic in the oil until golden. Sprinkle with ginger and stir. Add tomato and yogurt and a little water and cook uncovered until thickened. Add paprika. Add chicken pieces and cover. Simmer until almost done. Sprinkle with curry. Stir thoroughly. Remove cover and continue cooking until chicken is tender. If curry flavor is too strong, add a little milk.

SKIM MILK

Skim milk can be used as a substitute in any recipe calling for whole milk. It makes a refreshing drink.

BUTTERMILK

Buttermilk Biscuits
(1 doz.)

2 cups sifted whole wheat flour
½ t soda
1 t baking powder
½ C shortening
¾ C buttermilk
½ t sesame seeds
1 or 2 crushed rosemary leaves

Heat oven to 425 degrees. Sift together dry ingredients including rosemary. Cut in the shortening until mixture is crumbly. Add buttermilk gradually while stirring. Turn out onto floured board or counter and knead about ten times. Roll and cut into rounds. Sprinkle with sesame seeds. Place on baking sheets and bake about 14 to 15 minutes.

YOGURT

Yogurt Apple Salad

1 C yogurt
2 T honey
1 T lemon juice
½ C chopped raisins
½ C shredded coconut
3 big apples, finely chopped
½ C chopped nuts
Salad greens

Mix honey, lemon juice, raisins and chopped nuts. Fold in apples and yogurt. Spoon on greens for individual servings. Sprinkle with coconut. Serves 4.

Vegetable and Salad Dressing

1 carton plain yogurt
1 garlic clove, crushed
1 T grated onion
½ t dill or tarragon
½ t honey
½ t Worcestershire sauce
½ t Dijon mustard
freshly ground pepper

Blend all together. Chill. Will last several days in refrigerator.

Frozen Banana Yogurt

1 T unflavored gelatin
½ C water
2 large ripe bananas
2 C plain yogurt
¼ C honey
1 t vanilla
½ t cinnamon

Combine gelatin and water to soften. Heat at a low temperature until gelatin dissolves. Mash the bananas. Combine with yogurt, sugar, vanilla and cinnamon in blender jar. Whirl until well blended. Continuing to whirl, pour in gelatin until well blended. Pour into a bowl; freeze 1 to 2 hours until partially frozen. Stir once or twice, then beat until smooth. Return to freezer for 30 minutes. For smoother consistency, beat again. Spoon into sherbets or ice cream cones. Makes 4 to 6 servings.

DRIED MILK

Orange Cream Shake
(For one)

1 C chilled orange juice
½ C dried milk

Stir vigorously with a fork. Serve at once.

* * *

Dried milk can be blended with half the amount of water recommended and stored in refrigerator. Use directly in cream soups, milk drinks, desserts and custards. Do not boil in recipes as it will curdle.

Blender Fruit Pudding
(For 4)

Use 4 ripe peaches or
1 ripe papaya or other fruit in season
1 ripe banana
2 T dried milk
Honey to taste
Blend together and pour into bowls and chill thoroughly.

ACIDOLPHILUS MILK

Acidolphilus Milk can be used like yogurt and where not heated can be substituted in recipes calling for yogurt. For example, mix with some honey and use as topping for fruit or spoon a dollop on cucumber or other cold soups. It makes a delicious substitute for milk or cream in cold cereals.

COTTAGE CHEESE

Luncheon Cottage Cheese Loaf

1 C crushed pineapple, reserve juice
1 T gelatin
2 C cottage cheese
½ C grated carrots

In ½ C of the pineapple juice soak the gelatin. Simmer to dissolve. Add to the pineapple. Cool. Then add the carrots and cottage cheese. Stir well and chill to mold. Garnish with fresh mint leaves.

Cottage Cheese Pancakes

1 8 oz. container cottage cheese
1 container of yogurt
dash of ground cardamon (optional)
¼ C whole wheat flour
½ C chopped black walnuts

Add cottage cheese and honey to yogurt. Beat together. Add flour gradually. Drop by spoonfuls onto lightly greased griddle. Serve with more honey.

FARMER'S CHEESE

Farmer's Cheese can be used like other cheese. Place slices on top of vegetable casseroles or top sliced tomatoes on rye or whole wheat bread and broil until cheese is melted, not browned. High temperatures destroy some of its value.

CHEDDAR AND SWISS CHEESE

Cheddar Lentil Loaf
(For 4)

2 C cooked lentil beans
1 shallot or ½ small onion
1 small clove of garlic, pressed
1 C wheat germ
½ t thyme
Freshly ground pepper
1 egg, beaten
1 T oil

In blender or grinder mix cheese, lentils and onion and garlic. Season. Remove to greased baking dish and add rest of ingredients. Bake in moderate oven for 45 minutes. Serve with fresh tomato salad.

Rose May's Swiss Fondue
(For 4)

2½ lbs Swiss cheese
2½ lbs Gruyere
clove of garlic
pepper
nutmeg
1 bottle Leibfraumilch
2 - 3 t brandy or Kirsch
½ t cornstarch or arrowroot
whole-grain bread cut into chunks

Cut garlic clove in half and rub fondue pot. Sliver cheeses into pot. Sprinkle in some nutmeg and freshly ground pepper. Pour most of the wine. Heat only just before guests are to be served. Once fondue starts to melt, stir. Add the cornstarch and then the brandy. To eat, dip forkfuls of bread into the fondue.

LOW FAT CHEESES

Ricotta Pudding
(For 4)

¼ C grated Carob bar
½ lb ricotta cheese
¼ C finely chopped nuts
2½ T plain yogurt
½ t vanilla

Sprinkle the carob over the ricotta and blend until smooth. Stir in yogurt and vanilla. Serve in wine glasses.

RYE BREAD

Balkan Rye Bread
(2 Loaves)

2 T bakers yeast or 2 yeast cakes
½ C lukewarm water
4 T molasses or honey
1 large potato
4 T sesame oil
½ t iodized salt
5 C rye flour
2 C warm water

Dissolve yeast for 5 minutes in ½ C water. Stir in molasses. Peel and slice the boiled potato. Mash with its water through a sieve into a large bowl. Add oil and salt and the yeast mixture. Stir and then add 4 cups of flour. Beat together. Cover with towel dampened with hot water. Place in unheated oven. Put on oven light, close door and let stand for 1 hour. Now beat in the rest of the flour. Oil two bread pans. Divide dough into two parts and press into pans and smooth top with a little cold water. Put back into oven as before and let rise until bulk is about doubled. Bake at 375 degrees for about 45 minutes.

WHOLE WHEAT BREAD

Whole Wheat Honey Lemon

2 T yeast
2¼ C hot water
1 C dry milk
1 T salt
Rind and juice of one lemon
½ C honey
3 T butter
6 C(+) whole wheat flour

Dissolve yeast. Combine ingredients. Knead. Let rise. Form into 2 loaves in oiled pans. Let rise. Bake 40 minutes in 375 degree oven.

Whole Wheat-Honey Bread
(2 Loaves)

1 C milk
3 T oil
1 T salt

½ C honey

3 T active dry yeast

6½ C unsifted whole wheat flour

Optional

2 T molasses

½ C raisins

¼ C chopped prunes (dried)

½ C nuts (chopped) and/or

½ C sunflower seeds

Heat milk to simmer. Drop in oil, salt and honey (and molasses) into simmered milk. Add raisins and prunes to the hot milk. Pour into large mixing bowl. Cool to lukewarm.

Dissolve yeast in 1/3 C lukewarm water about 4 minutes. Add dissolved yeast to mixture in bowl.

Add 3 C flour. Stir 300 strokes by hand. Add 2 cups flour and stir well. Turn onto floured board. Knead until dough is smooth and firm, kneading in as much whole wheat flour as needed.

Place in oiled bowl, cover with warm damp towel and let rise in a warm place (80 to 85 degrees) for about 1 hour.

Knead down to original size, cover and let rise again.

Knead down to original size, shape into two or three loaves, place in oiled bread pans, cover with towel and let rise until dough begins to lift towel.

Preheat oven to 350 degrees and bake for 45 minutes, or until golden brown.

WHEAT BRAN

Bran Muffins

2 T yeast dissolved into

1 C warm buttermilk or water

3 T molasses

3 T oil

½ C raisins

1 beaten egg

1 C whole wheat pastry flour

1 C bran flakes

½ C wheat germ

½ C dried milk

1 t iodized salt

Dissolve yeast in liquid. Add egg, molasses and oil. Sift in remaining ingredients. Stir about 1½ minutes, adding raisins. Drop from large spoon into oiled muffin tins. Let rise in warm place until double. Bake for 20 minutes at 350 degrees.

* * *

Bran can be added to cereals, bread dough or other baked goods. When bran is added to your diet, drink an extra glass of water.

WHEAT GERM

Wheat germ can be added to all bread or cake doughs. It can be used to substitute for bread crumbs in most recipes. It can be added to cereals or eaten as a cereal. It can be cooked as a breakfast food as follows:

Wheat Germ Cereal

1 C skimmed milk
½ C wheat germ
½ t molasses or honey

Heat milk to simmer. Slowly turn in wheat germ and molasses. Cover and simmer about 5 minutes.

Wheat Germ Shrimp Loaf

2 C cleaned uncooked shrimps
½ C wheat germ
1/3 C dried milk
2 springs chopped parsley
1 garlic clove, minced
1 small onion, grated
½ t dill weed
freshly ground pepper
½ C dried milk
2 eggs
sesame or other salad oil

Oil shallow casserole dish and pack in mixture. Sprinkle with wheat germ and paprika and drizzle with a little oil.

TRITICALE
(See Chapter 3)

BUCKWHEAT

Mushroom Buckwheat Kasha

1 C buckwheat groats
2 eggs, beaten
1 C mushrooms, sliced
2 T oil (cold-pressed)
2 C water
2 cloves garlic, pressed
½ t Worcestershire sauce

Beat the eggs well and add the groats. Mix thoroughly. Brown mixture gently in oiled skillet. Add the sliced mushrooms and garlic. Boil water and add to the mixture. Add Worcestershire sauce. Mix well and cook very slowly, covered, until all the liquid is absorbed and the Kasha's fluffy.

Buckwheat Pancakes

½ yeast cake
¼ C warm water
¾ C boiling water
2 C buckwheat flour
2 eggs, beaten
1 cup dried milk
1 T molasses
4 T oil
¼ t soda
1 T molasses

Dissolve the yeast in the lukewarm water. Add 3 C boiling water to the buckwheat flour. When lukewarm, combine with the yeast and add all the ingredients except the last three. Cover with towels, set in a warm place, and let rise overnight. When ready to grill, add the soda dissolved in ¼ C boiling water and the molasses to the batter. Serve with maple syrup or honey.

SOURDOUGH BREAD

Starter for Sourdough

1 T yeast
½ C warm water
2 C warm potato water, diced and boiled with skins on
2 C whole wheat flour
1 T sugar or honey

Mix together and cover with towel. Let stand at room temperature from 2-4 days. Use glass or plastic, never metal bowl.

Sourdough French Bread

Using the Starter, place it in bowl with 2 T sugar, 2 C warm water and 1½ C whole wheat flour. Mix well and let stand at room temperature for 6 or more hours. Replace ½ C Starter in earthenware crock and refrigerate until needed again. Then repeat above step.

1 T yeast
1 T iodized salt (optional)
3½ C whole wheat flour
¼ C warm water
1 beaten egg to lighten dough (optional)

Dissolve yeast in warm water. Add it and flour to the Starter mixture. Turn out on floured board or counter and knead 25 times. Roll into a long loaf and sprinkle with cold water. Place in glass dish sprinkled with cornmeal. Let raise covered with damp towel until doubled. Bake at 350 degrees for one hour. During the baking, brush with water twice to get a glazed crisp crust.

Test for doubling: Poke 2 fingers into dough. If indent remains, dough has doubled. If it closes, let rise about 10 more minutes.

Hint: Flour hands to prevent dough from sticking when kneading.

SHREDDED WHEAT

Shredded Wheat Baklava

¼ C water
¾ C honey
2 t ground cinnamon
2 t grated lemon rind
6 Shredded Wheat Biscuits, split lengthwise
½ C margarine, melted
1 C chopped black walnuts
Whipped cream

Combine first four ingredients in a saucepan. Boil gently 15 minutes or until syrupy. Place Shredded Wheat halves in a single layer in a shallow baking pan; drizzle with margarine. Bake in a preheated moderate oven (375 degrees F) ten minutes, stirring once. Sprinkle half of the nuts over bottom halves of biscuits and drizzle with half of the warm syrup. Replace biscuit tops and drizzle with remaining styrup. Spoon excess syrup over biscuits until absorbed. Top with remaining nuts. Serve warm, topped with whipped cream. Makes 6 servings.

BROWN RICE

Rice Caribbean

1 C cooked brown rice
½ C dried apricots, cut fine
½ C currants or raisins cut in half
1 onion, chopped fine
2 or 3 rosemary leaves, pulverized
Quantro

Marinate the fruits, onion and spice in Quantro while rice cooks. When finished, stir in oil and a little butter or margarine. Toss with the marinated fruits.

Mushroom Rice With Tumeric
(For 4)

2 C mushrooms
4 T oil
½ C finely chopped onion
1 clove garlic, finely minced
½ t ground tumeric
1 C brown rice
1 bay leaf
1¼ C chicken broth
freshly ground pepper

Preheat oven to 400 degrees. Cut the mushrooms into cubes. Heat half the oil in a saucepan. Add the onion and garlic. Cook about two minutes and add the mushrooms. Cook about five minutes, stirring. Sprinkle with tumeric and add the rice and bay leaf. Stir until the rice is coated and add the chicken broth and pepper to taste. Cover and bring to boil. Then bake 20 minutes. Remove the cover and discard the bay leaf. Stir in remaining oil, while fluffing the rice.

Savory Rice Loaf

1 T oil
2/3 C chopped green pepper
1/3 C finely chopped onion
1 can (4 ounces) sliced mushrooms
½ C mayonnaise
4 C hot, cooked brown rice
2/3 C finely shredded Cheddar cheese
2/3 C wheat germ

1 t salt
1/8 t pepper
parsley

Melt margarine in small skillet. Add green pepper, onion, and mush-rooms. Cook over low heat, stirring frequently, just until tender.

Mix together mayonnaise, rice, cheese, bread crumbs, salt, pepper and sauteed vegetables in large bowl, tossing until well mixed. Press into 1 greased 9 x 5 x 3 inch loaf pan. Bake in 350 degree oven until well heated, about 30 minutes. Unmold onto serving platter. Garnish with parsley. Makes 6 servings.

WILD RICE

Cook 1 C wild rice in 1½ C soup stock.

Bring to boil, then cover and simmer 30 to 40 minutes or until tender. Season with freshly ground pepper to taste and ½ C finely minced onion and 3 minced fresh mushrooms.

BIRCHERMUESLI
(See Chapter 3)

OATS

Quick Oat Cereal

1/3 C rolled oats
1/8 C soy flour
¼ C sesame seeds
¼ C sunflower seeds
¼ C pumpkin seeds
raisins
1 t Brewers yeast
1 t calcium lactate powder
1 T wheat germ
1 T bran flakes
1 T honey
1 T dried milk

Mix all together in cereal bowl. Use buttermilk, acidolphilis or skimmed milk to moisten.

PASTA

Your Own Noodles

2 eggs
1/3 C dried milk
dash of iodized salt or kelp
whole wheat pastry flour

Stir together eggs, dried milk, salt and enough flour to make a stiff dough. Knead until pliable. Roll to thin. Let stand ½ hour. Cut into strips ¼ inch wide. They are now ready to boil.

ASPARAGUS

Asparagus In Milk
(For 3)

1 lb. asparagus
skimmed milk
parmesan cheese, grated
paprika

Heat enough milk to cover asparagus. Wash and break off asparagus stalks. Place carefully in hot milk. Cover and simmer about 9 minutes. Place on serving platter and sprinkle with cheese and paprika. Garnish with parsley.

BRUSSEL SPROUTS

Remove wilted leaves and split stems. Wash. Steam until tender. Place on platter and put small pat of margerine on top. Sprinkle over 1 T lemon juice and 2 T finely chopped toasted almonds.

SQUASH

Acorn or butternut squash should be split in half lengthwise. Remove seeds and fibers. Brush with margarine. Sprinkle with a little cinnamon and nutmeg. Cover with foil and bake ½ hour. If the squash is large, it should be quartered or it will require longer cooking.

CORN

Corn should be eaten as fresh as possible for maximum flavor. Take off outer husks. Leave at least one layer. Fold it back and remove silk and rinse. It can now be roasted in a hot oven for about 10 minutes or steamed on a rack for 3-4 minutes. Serve with margarine.

TOMATO

Tomatoes can be cooked in endless ways, but there is no greater thrill in eating than to pick a ripe tomato off a vine and eat it fresh. Even if store-bought, it is delicious in salads if added just before serving.

JERUSALEM ARTICHOKES

1 lb artichokes
1/3 C skimmed milk
fresh parsley
chives, chopped

Wash thoroughly. It is not necessary to peel the artichokes. Cut into halves. Heat milk. Drop in halved artichokes and stir until covered with milk. Cover and simmer until done, about 10 minutes. Sprinkle with chives and garnish with parsley.

ENDIVE
(For 4)

8 heads endive, halved lengthwise
¼ C oil
½ t dried basil
1 C consomme
4 T chopped black walnuts
1 T margarine
freshly ground pepper

Heat oil in large skillet and sprinkle in basil. Place the endives in skillet and season with pepper. Brown about 2 minutes per side. Add half of the consomme and simmer uncovered until tender. Add more consomme if needed.

Brown the walnuts in margarine. Place endive on serving platter and garnish with walnuts.

CALORIE-LESS FOODS

Three Bean Salad

½ green pepper
2 C cooked green beans
2 C cooked wax beans
2 C cooked kidney beans
¼ C honey

2/3 C vinegar
1/3 C vegetable oil
pepper to taste

Chop green pepper. Drain beans. Mix sugar, vinegar, vegetable oil, and pepper in a large bowl. Add vegetables. Mix well. Cover and chill at least 6 hours. Mix well before serving. Serves six.

KALE

Wash Kale and chop into large pieces. Steam without additional water a few minutes. Serve with a sauce made of Tahini (ground sesame), thinned with a little lemon juice.

OKRA

Okra and Tomatoes

1 C sliced okra
1 stalk diced celery
1 small onion
1 t grated parmesan cheese
½ C diced tomatoes
freshly ground pepper
pinch of dried basil or rosemary

Saute onion in a little oil with celery. Add rest of the ingredients and simmer about 10 minutes. Sprinkle with grated parmesan cheese.

BROCCOLI

Cut off thick stems, split and use for making soup. The rest of the stems can be split and steamed with the tops. Serve with cheese sauce made by dicing cheese and heating in milk or water. Add a little cornstarch, stirred into cold water first. This will keep the cheese a creamy consistency.

PUMPKIN

Pumpkin can be used, of course, as a pie filling. It also makes an excellent vegetable. Cook and serve like squash.

SWEET POTATOES

Sweet potatoes are at their most delicious when baked. Wash thoroughly. Cut off tips and wrap in foil. Cook at 375-400 degrees for 45 minutes to one hour, depending on size. For a company dish, mash and mix with fruit such as soaked apricots. Drizzle with orange juice and reheat.

SAUERKRAUT

Heat in a little water. Add 1 t caraway seeds or diced unpeeled apples with ½ t molasses and a dash of nutmeg.

ALFALFA

Alfalfa sprouts can be used to garnish soups, stews, salads. Use in sandwiches and spreads, in casseroles and meat loaves, scrambled with eggs. Add to breakfast dishes and use in high protein blended drinks.

GREEN BEANS
(See Three Bean Salad under CALORIE-LESS FOODS)

LENTILS

Grecian Lentil Soup

1 pkg. lentils
1 large onion, chopped
3 garlic cloves, chopped
2 stalks celery, chopped
6 canned plum tomatoes & juice
1 large bay leaf
4 springs parsley
¼ t dried mint leaves
¼ t dried basil
1/3 C olive oil
2 T apple cider vinegar
freshly ground pepper

Wash lentils. Cover with warm water and let stand for one hour. Bring to boil. Add onion, garlic, celery and tomatoes. Simmer, covered, one hour. Stir in herbs and oil. Simmer for another hour and a half until thick, stirring occasionally. Shortly before serving, add vinegar. Remove bay leaf and serve.

PEAS

One of the most common variety of vegetables. But have you ever tossed them raw in your salad?

CHICK PEAS

Peas Patties

Combine 1 cup chick peas with 3 cups cold water. Bring to boil and then simmer 2 minutes. Cover and let stand 1 hour. Cook peas in soaking liquid until tender. Drain and mash well. Combine with ½ cup minced onion and 1/3 cup minced green pepper. Season with salt and pepper. Shape into flat patties. Coat both sides with wheat germ. Fry in hot oil over medium heat until browned. Serve with meats or for breakfast.

MUNG BEANS

Purchase dried mung beans and sprout your own. Soak overnight in wide-necked jar. Next day, pour off all the water. Cover top of jar with piece of gauze or old nylon stocking held on by rubber band. Place at angle, propped up against edge of saucer. Rinse with fresh water a couple of times a day. Pour off water and replace as before. It should take 2-3 days for beans to sprout. Then refrigerate.

LIMA BEANS

Enchilada Bake

½ C dry limas, cooked with salt & pepper
1 onion, chopped
1 clove garlic, minced
5-6 mushrooms, sliced
1 green pepper, chopped
1½ C stewed tomatoes
1 T chili powder
1 t cumin, ground
½ C red wine
6-8 corn tortillas
½ C ricotta cheese and yogurt, mixed
black olives

Saute onion, garlic, mushrooms and pepper. Add beans, tomatoes, spices, salt and wine. Simmer gently for about 30 minutes. In an oiled casserole, put layer of sauce. Place tortillas on top. Garnish with cheese yogurt and the olives. Bake at 350 degrees for 15-30 minutes. Four servings.

ONIONS

Onions have been used in most of our vegetable recipes. Here is a recipe for small white onions.

Creamed Onions
(For 3)

9 small white onions
1½ T margarine

1½ T whole wheat flour
¾ C skim milk
freshly ground pepper
¼ C chopped parsley
dash of thyme

Cook onions in skin until tender. Drain and peel. Make cream sauce by melting butter, adding flour and stirring until mixed well. Add boiled milk and stir vigorously until thickened. Pour over onions. Sprinkle with seassonings.

GREEN PEPPERS

Vegetable Stuffed Peppers
(For 2)

2 medium green peppers
1 C cooked mashed soybeans
¾ T oil
1 T chopped onion
1 chopped garlic clove
½ C chopped black walnuts or cashews
2 t fine soy sauce
½ C grated cheddar cheese
¼ C tomato or lemon juice
½ C chopped celery or parsley
freshly ground pepper to taste

Remove seeds from peppers. Place them cut end down in a little boiling water and steam for a short time. Mix together all other ingredients. Fill peppers and sprinkle with paprika. Place in baking dish in which there is about ½ inch of water. Cover pan with foil or cover and bake in hot oven for ¾ of an hour.

CHIVES

Sprinkle over casseroles, into salads and sandwich fillings.

GARLIC

Garlic has been used in most of our recipes in this chapter.

RAW JUICES

A mixture of raw juices makes an excellent pick-me-up drink at the end of the day. Use regular juicer or prepare in your blender.

RAW FOODS

Japanese Salad

Using a hand or electric grater, grate a large slice of cabbage, ½ an apple with skin left on, ½ a carrot that has been scrubbed, 1 radish and 1 mushroom. Serve with favorite salad dressing.

FRUITS

Fruits such as APPLE, GRAPE, ORANGE, TANGERINE, GRAPE-FRUIT, PEACHES, PAPAYA (see Almond Chicken Salad recipe), AVO-CADO, BLACKBERRIES, PLUMS, PINEAPPLE, CHERRIES, STRAW-BERRIES, MANGO AND KIWIS are best eaten raw.

APRICOTS

Apricot Whip Au Rhum
(For 4)

1 C dried apricots
4 T honey
4 T dried milk
dash of rum or Quantro

Soak apricots with hot water to cover. Let stand for several hours. Place in blender with liquid. Add honey, dried milk and a dash of rum. Blend altogether and chill in wine or sherbert glasses.

WHEAT GERM OIL

Substitute wheat germ oil for olive oil or soy oil in making salad dressing.

PEANUTS

Peanuts are best eaten raw. That is, unroasted and unsalted.

CASHEW NUTS

Cashew nuts are also best eaten raw, unroasted and unsalted.

Cashew Salad Dressing

¼ C soy sauce
1 C cashews
½ t dill weed
½ t salad herbs

2 small cloves garlic
¼ C soy salad oil
½ C lemon juice
2 T honey

Put ingredients in blender with a small amount of oil. Blend until smooth. Add oil and water until dressing is thin enough to pour.

SESAME SEEDS

Sesame seeds can be eaten in the ground-form called Tahini. This is a nut-butter and is available in health food stores.

SOYBEANS

Soybeans should be soaked half a day in water, changing the water several times and then cooked in different water.

Soybean Macaroni Loaf

2¼ C cooked soybeans
¾ C whole wheat cooked macaroni
¾ T chopped onion
3 T oil
3 T whole wheat flour
1½ C milk
¾ C grated cheese

Combine oil, flour, and milk to make a white sauce. Add cheese and stir until melted. Combine all ingredients. Place in greased loaf pan. Bake 40 minutes at 350 degrees. Wheat germ and/or cheese may be sprinkled on top before baking. Serves 4 - 6.

BLACK WALNUTS

Black Walnuts can be substituted for any recipe calling for walnuts. Of course, they may also be eaten uncooked.

SUNFLOWER SEEDS AND PUMPKIN SEEDS

These seeds can be sprinkled on salads and into soups, used in casseroles and home-baked breads. See our recipe for Oat Cereal.

APPLE CIDER VINEGAR

Still popular with many health fans is the classic first-thing-in-the-morning-drink of equal parts of honey and apple-cider vinegar in the bottom of a tall glass, topped with plenty of water. Stir well. Can be made in large jar and kept in refrigerator indefinitely.

ACEROLA CHERRIES, CAMU-CAMU AND ROSE HIPS
(See Chapter 3)

POLLEN

A tablespoon full of pollen one-half-hour before a meal is an excellent way to maintain a high level of health. It can be mixed with honey and sun-dried, thus making a delightful candy. It can also be stirred into nut-milks.

AMINO ACID COMPOUNDS, BREWER'S YEAST
AND DESSICATED LIVER
(See Chapter 3)

BONE MEAL

Bone meal can be added to baked goods, cereals, stews and soups.

CAROB

See recipe "Ricotta Pudding" under Low Fat Cheeses. Carob can be in all recipes calling for chocolate.

BLACKSTRAP MOLASSES

See recipe for Rye Bread. Can be stirred into milk for a delicious night-cap.

LECHITHIN AND MINERAL WATER
(See Chapter 3.)

Chapter 8

Menus to Live by

Creating interesting ways to use "wonder" foods is fun. Putting them together for days of enjoyable dining is fun, too.

It is like a game of trying to sock as much vitality into a day's repasts as possible. How many "wonder" foods can I get into this meal and the next and into the snack in between? How can I pack in more protein? How can I cut animal fat, increase vitamins and minerals, while keeping the lid on calories?

It is a new way of culinary thinking and planning. It drops the old "sugar flakes, chocolate-covered twinkles" thought syndrome and substitutes the "chopped steak, salad" thought syndrome.

It is a switch from treating the taste buds and starving the body to treating the taste buds and feeding the body.

Food is a big subject. There used to be different foods in different areas of the country. Now, farm-to-market roads and express transportation give New York Florida oranges and give Florida New York's Littleneck clams. Fresh fish finds its way inland and the inland farm belt radiates its products all the way to the seacoasts.

Foods from other countries and other continents are becoming more common on store shelves. If not canned in syrup or doctored and preserved, they, too, become part of the ever-growing choices for our longevity menus,—sardines from Portugal, cheese from France and Switzerland, lamb from Australia.

As other countries become more affluent, they, too, enjoy international supermarkets. American and European food is now reaching Japanese tables in increasing variety.

At first, the results were expected to be healthier people. Indeed, the children started growing taller, but then tests showed that although the Japanese children were bigger than their predecessors, they were also weaker. They lacked strength, tired easily, were low in vitality, and had lowered resistance to disease. They tended to become obese. They lacked muscular coordination. There was more tooth decay and eyesight problems increased.

Can you imagine what sort of new imported American food the Japanese children were eating?

Fukutaro Takimoto, a 94-year-old farmer from Shikoku, Japan climbed the 12,000 foot Mt. Fuji in 1977 taking nine and a half hours. It was his third climb. He started at the age of 90 and expects to continue until 100. What kind of food do you think Farmer Takimoto has been eating?

"Imported" is not necessarily a stamp of approval on all food. We need to be selective in our use of this variety of food offered us from everywhere. We need to apply the protein-mineral-vitamin measuring gauges before we buy. And we need to be aware of how the food is packaged and preserved.

When you find a nutritious, new food, imported or domestic, put it on a list of options. We are creatures of habit in the supermarket. We tend to avoid the untried. Did you enjoy jellied madrilene at a friend's house for dinner? Put it on your option list. Take the option list along with your shopping list, so when you spot an option, you will remember.

Start your option list while reading this chapter. I will be mentioning dishes, combinations, and foods that may be new to you.

Capture the ideas for your upcoming eating variety and enjoyment. Option for a long life of culinary pleasure.

MENU PRINCIPLES TO FOLLOW

In the previous chapters, you learned about the basic principles behind the Longevity Diet. The sample menus that I present in this chapter are built on those principles.

Here are the major five building blocks of any Longevity Diet menu:

- It provides the necessary high protein requirements.
- It uses as many "wonder" foods as possible.
- It stays within moderate calorie limits.
- It minimizes animal fat and avoids sugar and other empty calories.
- It includes no foods with chemical additives, preservatives, or colorants.

The fourteen days of Longevity Diet menus in this chapter use the five building blocks.

Protein requirements are exceeded.

There are at least three "wonder" foods used everyday.

Calorie limits are observed for the average person consuming about 2,000 to 2,400 calories a day.

Vegetable oils, like margarine, are recommended instead of butter and no sugar or refined grains are used.

Fresh and frozen foods are called for, not canned or bottled. Where juices are on the menu, it is recommended that frozen juice or automatic juicers be used in preference to canned or bottled.

If you are scheduled for some weight loss before going on the regular Longevity Diet, the menus that follow can be used, providing the portions indicated are cut. A required 25 percent reduction in calories needs a corresponding 25 percent reduction in the size of portion.

Portions are measured in the most appropriate manner for the particular food. It can be by cup, tablespoon, or ounce. However, if no unit of measure seems appropriate, then the word "portion" is used, meaning whatever is considered to be a normal serving.

Watch your weight for the first week on the Longevity Diet, using these menus or your own. Should your weight show a tendency to rise, cut back on the portion. Smaller portions are usually just as filling and satisfying when protein and "wonder" foods are eaten because they are richer in nutrition and "stick to your ribs" in the no-hunger sense,—exactly the opposite of empty calories which keep you hungry while they stick to your ribs in the weigh more, live less sense.

Whenever a recipe is provided for the dish called for on a menu, an asterisk (*) indicates this. Refer to Chapter 7 under that "wonder" food to locate the recipe.

Here are 14 days of menus. They do not have to be used consecutively although some thought has been given to diversification and variety in the sequence shown. Also, leftovers are occasionally called for on a following day.

Leftovers are also good snacking. Two snacks are indicated for each day. Snack #1 is designed as a morning snack, snack #2 as an afternoon or evening snack. Place them where you want. Add snack times, if you wish, as long as weight remains constant.

The freedom of choice is yours. The pleasure is yours.

FOURTEEN SAMPLE LONGEVITY DIET DAYS

Day #1

Breakfast	½ cup pineapple chunks or crushed (in juice)
	8 oz. cup yogurt, plain
	1 slice whole wheat toast
	1 cup coffee
Lunch	6 tbs. tuna salad
	2 tbs. cottage cheese (low-fat)
	1 raw apple
Dinner	6 oz. roast leg of lamb (lean)
	1 cup cooked spinach
	1 portion salad, olive oil and apple cider vinegar
	½ cup banana-whip pudding
	1 cup herb tea
Snack #1	½ grapefruit
	1 cup Postum or coffee substitute
Snack #2	Raw peanuts, Chianti wine

Day #2

Breakfast ½ grapefruit
1 biscuit shredded wheat with milk and honey
1 cup Postum or coffee substitute

Lunch 4 oz. cold roast lamb
1 cup mung bean sprouts*
watercress
6 grapes
1 cup mint tea

Dinner 1 cup chicken consomme
1 portion chicken curry*
1 portion green peas
1 portion fruit foam*
1 cup coffee

Snack #1 5 oz. Acidolphilus milk

Snack #2 1 Bran muffin*
1 cup herb tea

Day #3

Breakfast 5 oz. orange juice
2 cottage cheese pancakes with honey
1 cup coffee

Lunch 4 oz. hamburger steak
1 grilled sliced onion
1 portion mixed greens with Roquefort cheese
dressing
1 cup herb tea

Dinner 4 oz. tomato juice
6 oz. halibut steak
1 portion lima beans
1 portion cole slaw
1 portion apricot whip au rum*
1 cup decaffeinated coffee

Snack #1 2 oz. quick oat cereal*
1 cup decaffeinated coffee

Snack #2 1 medium banana
1 cup herb tea

Day #4

Breakfast	1 medium raw apple
	2 eggs, any style
	1 medium slice toasted sourdough French bread*
	1 cup coffee
Lunch	4 oz. cold halibut
	1 portion cole slaw
	1 biscuit shredded wheat baklava*
Dinner	½ broiled chicken
	1 cup Jerusalem artichokes*
	1 portion Spinach salad
	1 cup gelatin dessert
Snack #1	5 oz. Acidolphilus milk
Snack #2	5 oz. frozen yogurt

Day #5

Breakfast	¼ medium cantaloupe
	3 buckwheat pancakes, honey
	1 cup coffee
Lunch	2 oz. sardines (Portuguese)
	1 cup yogurt apple salad*
	1 cup coffee substitute
Dinner	6 oz. sirloin steak
	1 portion broccoli
	1 portion alfalfa sprouts
	1 portion blender fruit pudding*
	1 cup herb tea
Snack #1	1 slice toasted sourdough bread with margarine
	1 cup decaffeinated coffee
Snack #2	¼ medium cantaloupe
	1 oz. pumpkin seeds

Day #6

Breakfast	1 cup orange cream shake*
	1 portion Birchermuesli with milk and honey*
	1 cup coffee

Lunch	1 portion wheat germ shrimp loaf*
	5 oz. Acidolphilus milk
	Celery and olives
Dinner	2 medium veal chops
	1 portion okra and tomatoes*
	1 portion gelatin dessert
	1 cup decaffeinated coffee
Snack #1	3 wheat thins and honey
	1 cup decaffeinated coffee
Snack #2	1 portion gelatin dessert
	1 cup herb tea

Day #7

Breakfast	2 medium tangerines
	3 oz. hamburger patty
	1 bran muffin
	1 cup coffee
Lunch	1 portion three bean salad*
	1 raw apple
Dinner	4 oz. turkey loaf
	1 portion endive*
	1 small yam
	1 cup raw fruit salad
	1 cup coffee substitute
Snack #1	2 oz. farmer's cheese
	1 cup decaffeinated coffee
Snack #2	2 oz. turkey loaf
	1 cup herb tea

Day #8

Breakfast	1 cup blueberries, milk
	2 eggs any style
	1 slice toasted sourdough French bread*
	1 cup coffee
Lunch	1 portion Swiss Fondue*
	1 portion mixed green salad
	1 cup frozen yogurt*

Dinner	4 oz. baked fresh salmon
	1 portion rice Caribbean*
	Celery stalks
	3 oz. pineapple chunks
	1 cup coffee substitute
Snack #1	5 oz. Acidolphilus milk
Snack #2	2 oz. cold salmon
	1 cup decaffeinated coffee

Day #9

Breakfast	5 oz. grapefruit juice
	1 portion bran cereal, milk, honey
	1 cup decaffeinated coffee
Lunch	1 portion almond chicken salad*
	5 oz. buttermilk
Dinner	1 portion Chinese steamed fish*
	1 portion mushroom rice with tumeric*
	1 raw green pepper, wedges
	1 portion ricotta pudding*
	1 cup coffee substitute
Snack #1	1 slice whole wheat honey bread*
	1 cup decaffeinated coffee
Snack #2	1 cup frozen banana yogurt*

Day #10

Breakfast	5 oz. orange juice
	3 oz. veal kidneys
	1 slice toasted whole wheat bread
	1 cup coffee
Lunch	1 portion soybean macaroni loaf*
	1 cup Japanese salad*
	1 cup herb tea
Dinner	2 shoulder lamb chops
	1 portion lima beans
	1 portion wild rice
	1 raw plum
	1 cup coffee substitute

Snack #1	5 oz. buttermilk
Snack #2	1 portion soybean macaroni loaf
	1 cup decaffeinated coffee

Day #11

Breakfast	5 oz. apple juice
	2 slices French toast (whole wheat), cinnamon, honey
	1 cup coffee
Lunch	1 cup cottage cheese
	1 sliced tomato
	1 portion watercress
	1 slice fruit cake (whole wheat)
	1 cup coffee substitute
Dinner	6 oz. beef stew
	1 cup Jerusalem artichokes*
	1 portion mixed green salad (Roquefort cheese dressing)
	1 portion strawberries
	1 cup herb tea
Snack #1	8 oz. skimmed milk
Snack #2	1 raw apple

Day #12

Breakfast	½ cup stewed rhubarb
	1 portion granola, milk, honey
	1 cup coffee
Lunch	1 cup lentil soup
	2 oz. cheese slices
	½ cantaloupe
Dinner	4 oz. calves liver with onions
	1 portion okra and tomatoes*
	5 oz. frozen yogurt
	1 cup coffee substitute
Snack #1	½ cup melon balls
	1 cup decaffeinated coffee
Snack #2	1 slice fruit cake
	1 cup herb tea

Day #13
Breakfast   ½ grapefruit
              2 oz. sardines
              2 slices Balkan rye bread* with margarine
              1 cup coffee

Lunch   1 portion creamed onions*
              1 portion raw chopped vegetables
              2 slices cheese
              1 cup herb tea

Dinner   6 oz. meat loaf
              1 portion string beans
              1 portion cole slaw
              ½ cup cherries
              1 cup decaffeinated coffee

Snack #1   Acidolphilus milk
Snack #2   2 oz. cold meat loaf
              1 cup coffee substitute

Day #14
Breakfast   5 oz. tomato juice
              1 portion quick oat cereal,* milk, honey
              1 cup coffee

Lunch   6 oz. asparagus in milk*
              1 slice fruit cake
              1 cup herb tea

Dinner   6 oz. roast sirloin of beef
              1 portion Brussel sprouts
              1 mixed green salad, oil and vinegar dressing
              1 portion melon
              1 cup coffee substitute

Snack #1   5 oz. buttermilk
Snack #2   2 cheese slices
              1 cup decaffeinated coffee

Bonus Menu
Breakfast   5 oz. grape juice
              ¼ cup bran cereal, milk, honey
              1 cup coffee

Lunch	1 large corn on the cob
	½ cup alfalfa sprouts
	1 peach
	1 cup herb tea
Dinner	7 oz. roast shoulder of veal
	1 portion cooked carrots
	1 portion spinach salad
	1 portion apricot whip au rum*
	1 cup herb tea
Snack #1	5 oz. Acidolphilus milk
Snack #2	2 oz. cold veal
	1 cup decaffeinated coffee

HOW TO SELECT THE MOST NUTRITIOUS MEATS

Meat is protein. But some meat has more protein per ounce than other meat.

The reason can be the density of the meat and the fat content. Meat with less fat content is usually denser meat for that reason, but there could also be water content.

The National Live Stock and Meat Board recently made a laboratory study of the calorie, protein, mineral and vitamin content of beef, pork, lamb and veal.

It showed that veal had more protein per ounce than the other three. It also showed that beef had more calories.

Here is what they found for a 3½ ounce portion of each:

	Beef	Pork	Lamb	Veal
Protein (grams)	29.6	28.5	26.6	32.7
Calories	265	240	258	213
Calcium (milligrams)	9.6	8.1	8.2	9.7
Iron (milligrams)	3.7	3.5	2	3.3
Phosphorus (milligrams)	191	228	211	260
Thiamin (milligrams)	.10	1.03	.22	.18
Riboflavin (milligrams)	.39	.29	.32	.35
Niacin (milligrams)	4.5	4.4	7.6	7.2
Vitamin B6 (milligrams)	.37	.46	.32	.48
Vitamin B12 (micrograms)	2.06	1.2	2.8	2.53

Veal is highest in four out of the nine categories. It is the lowest where lowness counts,—calories. So it has the best nutritional batting average.

Many people overlook veal in their menu planning. Savoury slices of roast veal can make any meal something special.

Your butcher can de-bone a leg of veal for you. Usually when he does this, and while tying it, he lards the veal with fat. Ask him not to lard it. And ignore that part of a recipe that tells you to cover the leg of veal with strips of salt pork or bacon. Also, go easy on any butter called for (use margarine), but you can go wild on the garlic, cloves and other spices.

A four-pound boneless leg of veal will take about two hours. When basting it, you might add a touch of dry white wine to the gravy. Later, when using the gravy, be sure to skim the fat off its surface first.

You can buy a breast of veal or a rump of veal and have it boned, too, for roasting. Or, you can buy veal chops or veal cutlets.

Veal chops can be baked, barbequed, or cooked in a covered skillet on top of the range. In the latter case, use wheat germ instead of bread crumbs for the coating. The same for veal cutlets.

When sliced into chunks or slivers, veal lends itself to a variety of gourmet dishes. Veal and peppers, veal paprika, veal stew and veal goulash are just a few.

Become more veal-minded. It is young beef that will help to keep you young.

Other meats are nutritious, too, but I won't give them equal time because they are probably more familiar to you.

If you like your beef rare, move a step in the other direction—to medium rare. Then try medium, perhaps later, even well done. You can train your taste. But you cannot train your arteries to ignore cholesterol.

A word about organ meats, though.

Liver is solid nutrition—chicken liver, calves liver, beef liver.

Also, brimming with minerals and vitamins are kidney, heart, brain and sweetbreads.

THE BEST OF POULTRY, FISH AND CHEESE

The best part of poultry is the liver. But chicken, guinea hen, squab and turkey are excellent protein. It is perhaps better protein than beef, pork, lamb and veal because it is less ingrained with animal fat.

You can control the fat more easily with poultry. It is usually confined to the skin and just inside the skin. Avoid eating the skin and you eliminate most fat. Also, white meat is leaner than dark meat.

Cooking melts fat. A duck is extremely fatty and should be over-cooked rather than under-cooked.

There are so many ways to cook chicken that it deserves a frequent place on your menu. Cold chicken is a good snack.

How many times a week? I would say at least once, but it is really a matter of taste.

Some authorities, for instance, say eat fish seven times a week. Fish is excellent protein, probably the best, but the increment is so small that a balanced, diversified diet seems to weigh more heavily. In other words, I prefer not to tell my clients to have certain foods so many times a week as long as "wonder" foods are given their full play.

Age, culture, race, location—all play a part in creating preferences. As long as these preferences are not subverted by sugar and processed foods, then a balanced diet of different proteins is fine. It's your choice.

A national columnist recently published a letter from an embarrassed wife whose husband was "hooked" on peanut butter sandwiches. He was turning down food offered by the hostess at a dinner or by restaurants and stuffing himself with peanut butter sandwiches instead. The advice was basically not to feel embarrassed, but to be concerned about the nutritional embarrassment of her husband.

Variety in menu planning is what counts. Don't get in a rut. Try new dishes.

Fish offers an even greater variety than do meat and poultry. Shellfish is a category by itself with a number of delicacies:

Soft shell crab	Mussels	Scallops
Oysters	Shrimp	Crayfish
Clams	Lobsters	King crab

Varieties of fish are endless. Fresh water fish are different than ocean fish and Atlantic Ocean fish are often different than

Pacific Ocean fish. Here is a reminder of some of the more common choices available to you in the fish market:

Bass	Herring	Shad
Bluefish	Mackerel	Smelts
Cod	Pike	Snapper
Eel	Pompano	Sole
Flounder	Porgy	Trout
Haddock	Salmon	Tuna
Halibut	Sardines	Whiting

And that is not all. Science is eyeing new oceanic resources. Species of fish exist that are not yet exploited. Ways may be found to utilize so-called bottom fish and "trash fish" that are caught and discarded. Squid are numerous and the catch can be 20 times if ways are developed to locate, harvest and prepare for market. Antarctica krill is the largest source of animal protein in the world and is untapped.

Fish can be baked, steamed, poached, barbequed and fried. In frying, again, avoid bread crumbs and use wheat germ.

Combine different fish in stews like the famous New Orleans bouillabaisse. Use shellfish for appetizers and snacks.

Most fish, especially shellfish, is not cheap, but if we as an affluent society must eat "rich" food, let it not be rich in butter, cream, pastry and sugar, but rich in the abundant minerals and nutrients from the sea.

Let's talk about cheese. It is seldom served at breakfast except perhaps in a cheese omelet, but it is prime menu choice for lunch, dinner and snacks.

When you shop, favor natural cheeses over processed. Look for imported cheeses especially because they pack more nutritional wallop per calorie. French Brie cheese is the original, American Brie the imitation. Ditto for Swiss Swiss over American Swiss. Blue cheese ranks low in nutrition compared to its French counterpart Roquefort, which is made from sheep's milk.

The people of Paris eat as much genuine Roquefort in a year as the whole United States. There are other veined cheeses like it from abroad—Britain's Stilton and the Danish Blue.

Traditional European cheeses are produced in rural areas

from animals that graze and by time-consuming, old-fashioned methods.

What that should say to you is no chemicals and lots of "wonder" nutrition.

The key for cheese-lovers is "low-fat". Let this be your over-riding guide.

HEALTHFUL COMBINATIONS OF GRAINS, FRUITS AND VEGETABLES

As you see by the 14 sample days Longevity Diet menus, either a fruit or a vegetable is in every meal. And where a grain is used, it is a whole grain.

Menus need to recognize the local availability of fruits and vegetables in fresh or frozen form. If a canned or bottled fruit must be used, it should be rinsed of its syrup.

Vegetables can be generally classified as leafy or starchy. The starchy variety can be further divided between those that grow above ground and those that grow below ground.

The order of low calorie - high nutrition is:

(1) Leafy green
(2) Leafy, white
(3) Starchy, above ground
(4) Starchy, below ground

Every daily menu should include (1) at least once, in the raw state. Examples are: green lettuce leaves, spinach, watercress, parsley.

Every other day would be a respectable frequency for (2). Examples are cabbage, endive, and artichokes.

The starchy above ground vegetables come in lesser and greater degrees of starch. String beans and snow peas have less starch than lima beans and green peas. Go by the pulpiness of the product. Once every few days would be a proper frequency for (3), with the less starchy beans favored.

Again with (4), we have varying degrees of starchiness. I would exempt carrots from frequency control, but at the other end of the spectrum I would place beets, potatoes and sweet potatoes under strict control.

In fruit, the sweetness appears to be the controlling factor. Citrus fruits—oranges, grapefruit, tangerine—are generally good nutrition per calorie. Apples are excellent, the more tart the better. It is when you get into the plums, nectarines, and grapes that the fruit sugars begin to add up.

Melons such as cantaloupe are fine. The sweeter honeydew and watermelon are to be quantity and frequency controlled. Blueberries, strawberries, blackberries, and raspberries are worth grabbing for your menus when in season.

The criteria for grains is how natural and how cooked. Grains baked in bread and muffins are not damaged as badly as grains cooked in dry cereals. Natural brown rice, though considered by Oriental peoples not to have as much prestige as white rice, has triple the nutrition.

Wheat is probably the only other grain that is tampered with. Oats, barley and corn usually come in natural form.

Grains make good breakfasts and good desserts.

LONG LIVE DESSERTS!

Desserts are probably the greatest curse to man's nutrition, but have become the most ingrained.

We reward ourselves with desserts. We top off our meals with desserts. We snack with desserts.

The crowd that shouts "Long live desserts!" will live longer themselves without them.

However, there are plenty of desserts that are not a curse, and instead can be a nutritional blessing.

Chocolate is a curse. Even in its non-sweetened form, it leeches vitamin C. Use carob in its place.

Whole grain carob cookies and cake are acceptable desserts if you do not add too many eggs, too much shortening and too much sweetening to the batter.

Honey is the favored sweetener, but pure maple syrup comes in a close second. Beware of imitation maple-flavored syrups which are largely sugar and other "pancake" syrups.

Create your own desserts from "wonder" foods. Think in terms of fruit, seeds, and nuts.

Good bases are cottage cheese, dry milk, and gelatin.

The home blender is a useful dessert tool. Raw apple slices when blended become apple sauce. Banana when blended becomes a whip. Other fruits blended become interesting dessert puree.

Skin bananas, freeze them, then put them through the blender and you have banana "ice cream." You can do this with other fruits, too.

The white of egg can be used interestingly as meringue. Avocado whipped with lemon and honey is a tasty dessert. Zabaglione made with egg yolks is alright if you have not used up your quota (2) for the week. It is made with honey and Marsala wine.

A touch of wine and a touch of rum add interest to many desserts where sugar leaves a vacuum.

Whipped cream has very few calories and adds a party look to desserts. Use it as a garnish, not as the main ingredient.

A reminder: vitamin and mineral supplements may not appear on your menus, but they should be on your shopping list. Vitamins E, C, and B-complex are priority. Any multi-mineral supplement (organic) is helpful.

HOW TO EAT AT A PARTY WITHOUT PENALTY

What happens when you go to somebody's house for dinner and have no say in the menu? If this happens frequently, you have a problem. If it happens once a month or less, it is a very minor matter.

In either case, you go easy on the fatty food and on the sweets and starches. You make up for it on the protein and on the vegetables and fruits. The more frequently you accept dinner invitations, the more conscientious you need to be in your selection.

The same applies at restaurants. Enjoy fish or meat appetizers; fish, poultry, or meat entrees; salads; but only fresh fruit or low-fat cheese desserts. Ignore the white bread that is put in front of you.

Then there are the hors d'oeuvres at cocktail parties. Look for the cheese cubes. Take a toothpick and spear a meatball.

Monopolize the shrimp (without the dip). Avoid the canapes or open sandwiches unless you are skilled at stealing the caviar or other topping off with your teeth and dumping the bread or cracker where it belongs—the garbage.

At your own party, be creative when you make the cocktail snacks. Use protein and "wonder" foods. It will be a better party.

Put out raw cauliflower with a cheese dip. Serve green pepper slices with an onion dip.

Broil prawns and serve them with mustard. Stuff mushrooms with cheddar cheese. Mix chopped beef with ground ginger and soy sauce for meat balls and bake them in a slow oven. Put out hard-boiled whites of eggs stuffed with asparagus; serve lamb kebabs that the guests can cook themselves; cut wedges of melon with thin slices of prosciutto ham.

The choice is endless in whatever direction you choose to go. If you go shortevity, serve a Viennese table of fancy cream pastries. If you go longevity, serve a table replete with such seafood, meat, cheese, and fruit goodies that your guests will not stop talking about it all your longer living days.

THE SMART WAY TO DRINK
AT A PARTY OR BUSINESS LUNCH

Unfortunately, whenever people get together socially, liquor seems to be a feature. If you are a good drinker, you are the life of a party. Even business executives are often judged by their alcoholic strength.

Recently, it was found in actual field tests that given a tiny drink of alcohol used in a spray, the response was higher yields of corn, cucumbers and other crops.

We respond, too, with tiny drinks. But we don't stop there, and as we continue to drink in the interests of society, our own health interest goes down the drain and the results are often disasterous for both the evening and the long run.

You can keep up the look of being a good drinker without making a fool of yourself. There are a few tricks you can use. It is the smart way to drink.

Here are some examples:

- Use a large glass instead of a small one, but with the same amount of liquor. Talk with it in your hand. Gesture with it.
- Sip slowly, using your hand on the glass to conceal how small a sip you really take.
- Drink straight drinks and drink what does not taste good to you. Avoid even lemon if it makes it taste better.
- Pace your drinks. One shot an hour is the limit the average weight person can take without exceeding the body's capacity to purify the blood.
- Become a connoisseur of wine or scotch or other liquor. "Talk" a good drinker.

You can live it up at parties without cutting down on your life.

PREPARING TO EXTEND YOUR LONGEVITY STEPS

This concludes the basic Longevity Diet, but it is only the beginning of the steps you can take to prolong your life.

In the next chapter we will talk more about food, but from a weight normalizing point of view. Add pounds and you subtract years.

Studies show that in the past ten years men and women have averaged a weight gain of a pound or two up to 14 pounds, depending on height, despite all the attention to reducing pills and exercise salons.

This is not true in Yugoslavia, for instance, when the oldest citizen, Mrs. Jovanka Vasiljevic, aged 120, has been found growing a new set of teeth. She recently was the guest of honor at the first convention of Yugoslav gerontologists, escorted by her 81-year-old son.

Affluence in America is costing us longevity. In Chapter 9, we learn how to shed costly pounds quickly, easily, and permanently.

But, we do not cease our attack on shortevity there.

"Better to eat a dry crust of bread with peace of mind than have a banquet in a house full of trouble," says the Bible in Proverbs 17:1. We have known for millennia that stress can render the best nutrition worthless. It is time we did something about it.

In Chapter 10 we cover special diets to give us more energy to handle stress and to function at a higher sexual level,—a prime stress factor.

In Chapters 11, 12, and 13, we take aim at specific stress factors and acquire mental techniques to insulate ourselves from them. We examine other health enemies and acquire weapons to combat them. And we learn ways to control our minds that can add years to our lives.

Chapter 9

Slimming Down for Longer Life

We have prepared for a longer life.

We have shifted our foods away from fats and starches. We have added in their place proteins and foods bursting with vitamins and minerals. We have identified and blackballed the chemicalized and denatural foods.

We have reorganized our menu planning along protein and caloric guidelines, and we have acquired recipes that utilize the "wonder" foods.

If you have been "gung ho" for better health, more energy, and a longer productive life ahead of you, you probably began to avoid sugar and white flour in Chapter 1. By now you have tried many of the "wonder" foods and have been emphasizing body-renewing protein in your daily fare. You may even have tried a recipe or two.

You need not wait another day. In fact, you should not wait another day. Swing into the Longevity Diet all the way, today.

Every day's delay is another day on the Shortevity Diet.

You have all the information you need to begin. There are other actions you can take. I am going to tell you about these in the chapters ahead, but I want you to understand that these are not pertinent to the Longevity Diet per se. Begin the Diet. Begin it today.

These other actions begin with this chapter. If you are overweight, this chapter concerns you. But still you do not have to wait. You already have weight reduction menus alongside the weight maintenance menus in Chapter 7. Even if you are not overweight, you will still want to have the information in this chapter should you be faced with the problem in the future.

In subsequent chapters we will review special diets for special problems. We will also learn how to cope with the dangers of stress and of the sedentary life—two more health-sapping factors of modern living. We will learn techniques for using our minds to keep us well, reversing the psychosomatic causes of disease.

Now let's take a look at these extra pounds.

ANATOMY OF AN OVERWEIGHT PERSON

Perhaps I just said the wrong thing. No chubby person likes to look at the extra flab. But this excess baggage is loading you down. I don't mean just more weight to carry for your legs. It is loading down your liver. It is an extra load on your kidneys. It is loading down your heart.

Extra pounds require your body to do so much extra work that not even "wonder" foods can balance the years lost from your life.

Extra pounds cost years. There is no way to erase that fact. To save your life, you must lose those pounds.

Let's really take a look at those pounds. A full-length mirror tells the story even better than a scale. Especially if we stand in front of it naked. Take your clothes off. Do it now.

Stand facing the mirror. Look at yourself straight in the eyes. Without changing your gaze, are you aware of aspects of your face that betray extra flesh on cheeks or chin? Now direct your gaze to those parts. Confirm what you suspected. Look intently at the cheeks, chin. or neck—wherever you became aware of tissue excess.

Continue down your body to arms, chest, stomach. Each time you halt your gaze on a guilty portion of the anatomy, acknowledge the excess and become aware of the next part of your body that deserves attention even before you move your eyes.

The stomach is a prime location for unwanted blubber. Take your two hands and grasp the outer layers. Does it form handfulls? These handfulls are you. They are alive. They are not essential to your life. They are borrowing their life from the life of organs that are essential to your life.

Check your hips, thighs, knees, legs. Identify. Acknowledge.

Now, before you turn and see yourself from a sideways angle, imagine how you will look. Are there extra pounds on your back and buttocks? Now turn and look. Inch around just a bit more so you can see part of your back. Confirm. Identify. Acknowledge.

Extra pounds sneak in. They put a foot in the door and if you don't slam the door, the rest of them tiptoe in. They are there by tacit agreement. You don't like to talk about that pound on your knee, that pound on each of your upper arms. But now your tacit agreement is about to change to an affirmation of disagreement.

Before you can lose weight, you must agree to do so. You must disagree to gain more weight and you must disagree to provide a home for the excess pounds you have now identified.

Right this minute—standing there in honest nudity—make that affirmation. The words could be: "I recognize the excess pounds I carry. They sap my vitality and shorten my life. I now decide to normalize my weight and lengthen my life."

Close your eyes. See yourself thin. The slenderizing process has begun.

ADVANTAGES OF THE LONGEVITY DIET IN LOSING WEIGHT

In the introduction to this book, I described how I discovered the basic Longevity Diet while observing my weight-loss clients. The weight-loss diet was not only succeeding in slenderizing them, but they were staying youthful and attractive year after year on the maintenance diet.

The Longevity Diet is a weight maintenance diet. The Longevity Diet with only a few minor changes is a weight loss diet, and a "painless" one at that.

Step One in losing weight is to go on the Longevity Diet and enjoy this nutritious change.

If you are seriously overweight, 50 pounds or more, you may even begin to lose weight on the Longevity Diet. But this is not the purpose of Step One. The purpose is to make the transition to weight loss a small one.

Most diets fail because the diet is so different. You give up all your favorite foods and go on totally unsatisfying foods. This is not such a diet. In fact, you will hardly change any foods at all.

Step Two in losing weight is to prepare to reduce the size of portions of certain foods—these will be foods high in fat, like cheese, and high in carbohydrate, like fruit. More about this later in this chapter.

Step Three in losing weight is to add a couple of meals. Yes, in return for cutting certain portions, you are going to enjoy as many as five or six meals a day as you lose.

So once you are on the Longevity Diet, all you do is cut certain portions and add meals. Do not expect to suffer one single hunger pang. Do not expect to sacrifice one iota of eating pleasure.

Sound too good? Well, ask any one of thousands who have slenderized on my weight loss plans. No sweat. No tears. No failure.

Take Mrs. Marilyn M. When she first came to my office some ten years ago, she was a cake-aholic. She would go on a bakery binge every few days. She would bring home her loot and have it for breakfast, lunch, dinner and in-between. In her early thirties, she looked 40. She admitted that her 169 pounds now interfered with her favorite sport tennis and she seldom went on the courts. She did not have enough energy to move her weight around.

Substituting high protein foods for breads, rolls, cakes, pies, and cookies, Marilyn was able to shift to a lower calorie intake without hunger. Hamburger steak, they say, "sticks to your ribs" for longer because it takes longer to digest. That is true. But the hamburger rolls actually stick to your ribs as fat, maybe forever, albeit creating a shorter forever.

It took some maneuvering with Marilyn to make the switch. I appealed to her outdoors nature and had her try pheasant, then keep leftover slices and bones as between-meals snacks. I appealed to the "good sport" in her to try veal kidneys, sweetbreads and other organ meats she had been "chicken" to try before. I appealed to the gourmet in her and suggested she try Bouillabaisse and new types of shellfish for her, like mussels.

I suggested things she could do with a large primal rib to save money as she lost pounds. I told her how to go to the meat counter in a supermarket if she did not have a local butcher, ring the bell and tell the butcher she would like to buy a whole beef rib and have it "hung back" for a couple of weeks of aging. I warned her he might say he does not have a rail to hang it on, or that it is against his company's policy, but then again he might smile at her appreciation of a good standing rib.

Most markets do not age ribs any more. Either they do not have the rails to hang them on, or their refrigerator space is full of fast moving meat. So the ribs remain wrapped in plastic and packed in boxes on the floor where they do not age to perfection.

If the butcher agreed, Marilyn was to select a whole rib, about 25 pounds, well covered with white fat, a necessity to proper aging. Of course, the fat will cause us to age, too, so it is later trimmed off. The butcher will cut the rib down to seven inches, shorter than the usual ten inches, but best for a standing roast. At Marilyn's request, he will also remove the "chine" bone and cut off a few ribs as steaks for freezing. The standard primal rib contains seven ribs. Allowing two persons to a rib, you can figure how many ribs to cut off as steaks.

What I was really doing was involving Marilyn in a food adventure, exciting enough to eclipse her propensity for the bakery.

There is a big difference between the butcher and the baker. If you must have an affair with one, it will last longer with the butcher.

Being a cake-aholic, Marilyn had to be off that stuff completely. One bit and she was a goner. The steaks and roasts did the trick. Marilyn lost weight steadily while she enjoyed filet mignon, rib steaks, roast prime rib and chopped steak.

That was her main switch—baker to butcher. Three years later Marilyn weighed a sylph-like 107 pounds and was a whiz once again on the tennis courts. Now, seven years later, she looks younger than when I first saw her.

The Longevity Diet is more permissive than the weight loss diet in some ways.

HOW TO DESTROY FAT
WHILE YOU FEED YOUR BODY WELL

Dr. Sarfaraz Niazi, Associate Professor of Pharmacy at the University of Illinois Medical Center in Chicago, made an interesting discovery quite by accident. He was experimenting with a chemical called perfluoroctyl bromide on test animals to see if it could help in cases of overdoses of aspirin and barbiturates by coating the stomach and preventing absorption.

It worked. But Dr. Niazi noticed also that the test animals lost a significant amount of weight during the experiments. Apparently, so well does the drug coat the gastrointestinal tract that it temporarily blocks food absorption.

"The dieter's dream" is the way the press handled the news. But that dream can well become a nightmare. If the Food and Drug Administration approves the use of this chemical—and it must first reaffirm that it does not enter the bloodstream or accumulate in vital organs like the liver, gallbladder, spleen or muscles—then people who lose weight will be starving their body to do so.

Just to get mouth satisfaction, they will be risking injury to vital organs through cutting off vital nutrients. It is about as unnatural an act as you can think of.

On the other hand, losing weight on the Longevity Diet is about as natural a way as you can think of.

It feeds your body on top priority protein, vitamins, and minerals. Not one cell starves, so how could you possibly be hungry. Plus there is mouth pleasure galore.

Here is the meat of why the Longevity Weight Loss Diet works:

1. Carbohydrates slow down the metabolic rate. Proteins speed up the metabolic rate. You burn more calories on proteins. You store more calories on carbohydrates.
2. You can eat more proteins than carbohydrates calorie for calorie and still lose weight. However, the carbohydrates act as "hooks" to hang the weight on you. They must be carefully controlled.

Rubner discovered in the late nineteenth century, that a man metabolized 2,566 calories a day on meat, but only 2,450 calories on sugar. A 2,500 calorie diet of meat was a weight-loss diet. The same calories of sugar was a weight-gain diet.

For generations doctors were telling their overweight patients "Get off sweets and starches." Now we seem to have forgotten this fact. So we starve on a rice diet or struggle along on melba toast and carrot sticks.

Such suffering is not necessary. Protein keeps your metabolic fires going; you can eat plenty of gut food, while you fully nourish your slenderizing body.

The high protein foods on your Longevity Diet are the fat-destroyer foods on your Longevity Reducing Diet.

CUTTING PORTIONS TO CUT WEIGHT

Because proteins destroy fat, they will come under less scrutiny as we now prepare to turn the Longevity Diet into a Longevity Weight-Loss Diet.

The only protein portions we will want to cut are those proteins with sizeable fat content.

This means if fat is marble-ized throughout a cut of beef, you need to cut that portion in half. You need to be extra conscientious about trimming fat off beef. You need to cook the meat a bit longer than you prefer to if your taste goes for rare or medium rare.

You need to be conscientious about avoiding poultry skin, and you need to cut your portions of dark meat. You can have your usual portion of white meat.

Eggs are another source of fatty protein. Egg yolks contain substantially more cholesterol than any other common food. They are a major contributor of cholesterol in the American diet.

As you saw in Chapter 4, the Longevity Diet recognizes this by limiting egg yolks to two a week. I am not asking you to cut this, but I am asking you to observe this limit conscientiously if you are on the Longevity Weight-Loss Diet. How about buying the medium eggs instead of large?

Egg producers have been advertising that there is no increase in heart and circulatory diseases among people who eat eggs. This was intended to counteract a steadily declining per capita egg consumption due to the cholesterol-content publicity. However, now the Federal Trade Commission has prohibited egg ads from claiming there is a lack of scientific evidence linking eggs with heart disease.

In my opinion, the only aspect of this question left in doubt is: How much harmful cholesterol is manufactured by the body itself? Some people manufacture their own cholesterol in excessive amounts and can develop circulatory problems without ingesting any cholesterol to speak of. But whatever the ultimate answer to that question, the person desiring to lose weight should eat less fat. That means fewer egg yolks.

Cut cheese portions in half. Watch every drop of salad oil, every pat of butter. And remember—shortening means life shortening. These are also sources of fat that, unless monitored, can throw calorie counts out of whack and cause the pointer on your scale to take off.

The real portion cutting must come in the grain, fruit and vegetable categories.

Eat less bread—limit yourself to one slice a day. Eat smaller portions of cereal—half of usual. Cut rice portions a little, but cut pasta and noodles out altogether until your weight-loss goals are reached.

Fruit contains fruit sugar. It is not as life shortening as cane sugar. But the carbohydrates in fruit are the hooks on which fat can hang.

While you are losing weight, you must keep a wary eye on fruit. Some are low in fruit sugar. No problem. But others are quite high. To help you know the difference, I have placed the common fruits into three categories: "OK," "1/2 Portion," and "No."

OK	1/2 Portion	No
Rhubarb	Orange	Avocado
Cantaloupe	Pineapple	Apricot
Strawberries	Apple	Fig
Grapefruit	Pear	Raisin
Raspberries	Plum	Grape

Peach	Nectarine	Cherry
Tangerine	Watermelon	Prune
	Honeydew Melon	Banana
		Persimmon
		Date
		Kumquat

By now, there should be no need of my saying "fresh not canned." If canned or frozen, it should be water packed and no sugar added.

Now let's do the same for vegetables.

OK	1/2 Portion	No
All calorie-less "wonder" foods	Carrots	Potato
	Onions	Peas
Soy beans	Beets	Kidney beans
Cabbage	Artichoke	Lima beans
Lettuce	Eggplant	Corn
Kale	Broccoli	Sweet Potato
Celery	Turnip	Lentils
Tomato		Dried beans
Radish		

A good rule to follow is: the leafier the better, the pulpier the worse. Above ground growth seems to produce fewer carbohydrates than below ground. However, soy beans seem to be a pulpy bean, but it is a "wonder" bean in that it is almost 100 percent protein.

Again, canned is an inferior choice to fresh. Frozen is better than canned but not as nutritious as when you cook fresh vegetables with minimum water.

Now let me reward you for cutting those portions.

THE SAME AMOUNT OF FOOD
IN MANY MEALS IS BETTER THAN IN ONE MEAL

So far, I have not asked you to starve. There are scores of foods you can eat all you want. I have asked you to cut portions of certain foods like bread, oils and fat.

You do need some oil. Oils have a way of decreasing hunger. They retard the emptying time of the stomach. A little oil, as on salad, should be taken everyday.

Potatoes are about the only food you might miss. However, it is only temporary. Potatoes are calorie-high. But they pose no other threat to longevity. So, once your weight is normal, you can return potatoes to your fare.

Many dieters follow a familiar pattern. They skip breakfast, eat a light lunch, then eat a large dinner. Some of these dinners begin with cocktails at 5 p.m. including snacks, and then after the main event continue with drinks and snacks until midnight.

What they are doing is loading their fuel supply with an excess. That excess must be stored as fat. They are doing this prior to sleep when the body burns less fuel than during waking hours. It is about the worst way to handle your fuel supply.

Have you ever watched herbivorous mammals eat? Or birds? It appears that they eat almost constantly. They are really having 12 small meals a day instead of our three square meals a day. Their weight is never a problem.

When food is converted into fuel for immediate use, it need not be stored. The storing process is the gain weight process.

Six 300-calorie meals can produce weight loss for some people, while three 600-calorie meals can cause these same people to gain. The total calores is the same 1,800, but the need to store those calories, even for a few hours, gets that conversion process going, a process that we do not want to get started.

We average about 200 calories burnt off an hour, more during waking hours, less during sleeping hours. Ideally, it would be less-fat producing if we could eat our meals with this in mind.

Of course, we cannot all eat like sparrows. But it is better to eat constantly like a sparrow, taking in what we need, than like a vulture, taking in everything that's there.

Less than a decade ago, Dr. P. Fabry, head of the Physiology Department of the Institute of Human Nutrition in Prague, Czechoslavakia, reported that he found that men patients who ate three square meals a day tended to become overweight as compared to other men patients who ate five or more smaller meals. He also found that these three-square-meal men had impaired blood sugar levels and high cholesterol levels by 60 to 64 years of age. Over 30 percent had ischemic heart disease while less than 20 percent of the patients who ate five or more meals a day suffered from the heart ailment.

Dr. Fabry did not claim he knew why this was so. Did the big meals cause it or did the small meals prevent it? The important fact was that five or more smaller meals a day proved to be a healthier way of life than three bigger meals.

So even you normal-weight folks can borrow a page from this chapter.

But, herein lies a boon to the overweight. Divide up your weight-loss meals into two installments and you can eat more and keep losing the same amount, or eat the same amount and lose more.

If you time these meals so that the energy they provide is available when it is needed, you are further reducing the likelihood that your fat-storing processes will be called upon.

Figure on a lead time of three hours. It takes about three hours for food, once it enters the mouth, to become energy.

You need a substantial breakfast to provide midmorning energy supplies. But you do not need a big dinner to go to sleep on, nor do you need that late evening or midnight snack.

The Longevity Diet foods are going to keep you better nourished on half the food than your quickie-food neighbors on twice the food.

HOW TO ADD MEALS AND SUBTRACT POUNDS

I recommend that you plan on two breakfasts, two lunches and one dinner. This means dividing your breakfast menu in two parts and doing the same with your lunch menu.

This might be a typical day's menu:

Breakfast #1 (7 a.m.)	Breakfast #2 (10 a.m.)
Half grapefruit	American cheese
Granola and skim milk	Wheat thins
Decaffeinated coffee	Skim milk

Lunch #1 (noon)	Lunch #2 (3 p.m.)	Dinner (7 p.m.)
Tuna salad	Chicken leg	Roast beef
Herb tea	Yogurt	Spinach
		Salad
		Gelatin dessert
		Decaffeinated coffee

Approximate calories (average portions):   1,600

If you are a late person, you might want to have your gelatin dessert a couple of hours after dinner when you watch a late movie on television. However, remember that the storage mechanism is triggered by too much food eaten too close to bedtime.

In preparing your Longevity Weight-Loss Diet menus, you need to keep in mind the Longevity Diet guidelines:

1. Stay above minimum protein requirements.
2. Stay below maximum caloric allotments.
3. Favor "wonder" foods.

Then you add these Weight-Loss guidelines:

4. Cut portions.
5. Add meals.

In South Africa, there are aborigines who depend largely on wild game for their survival. They are called the Hottentots. When they make a kill, they have no way of storing the meat, so they must devour it all at one "sitting." It might be their last meal for three days. Can you imagine what a Hottentot looks like? Imagine a body that must store fat. If you picture mounds of fat on the Hottentot, you are right. The camel stores for the days ahead in a hump on his back. The Hottentots have humps of fat round their buttocks.

The camel's hump does not go away. It remains on standby. Same with the Hottentot. Same with you. A Yale University psychologist and obesity expert recently reported her research findings to the American Psychological Association. Fatness can breed fatness she said. "Being fat can keep you fat. If you have enlarged fat cells from gaining weight, your body is primed to store more of what you eat as fat."

You have already discovered your "humps." Gear your eating to your energy needs. Stay at that level, and you will not have to carry these "humps" around forever.

DIETETIC FOODS
HAVE CALORIES TOO ... PLUS

"What about diet foods?" I am constantly asked. "Are they permitted?"

This is a complicated question. Some so-called diet foods have no fewer calories than their non-diet counterparts. Others contain substitute sweeteners that might be less than healthful.

To sacrifice years of your life to lose pounds from your body is like throwing the baby out with the bath water.

There is a firm on the island of Maui in Hawaii that packs pineapple for most of the private-label brands offered by major chains. They use the exact same product for every label. In an interview with the *Enquirer* recently, a sales representative for the Maui Company explained how the only difference really is price. "Diet" pineapple chunks cost 75 cents, while regular supermarket brand chunks cost 59 cents. They both have the same number of calories.

It was also found that green beans on a brand label that says "For sodium and calorie-controlled diets" has the same calorie content as national-brand green beans. Some so-called dietetic sandwich cookies have even more calories than familiar makes and cost more.

A dietetic cheese thin has five calories per gram compared to four calories per gram in a well-known non-diet brand and cost 40 percent more.

I am not condemning all so-called diet foods by the misrepresentations of a few, but I follow the same basic precept in diet as I do in Longevity: Control your own food. Do not let others process it, cook it, color it, or doctor it.

In this way, you control your own calories, too. All of the controversy over saccharin and other artificial sweeteners makes it all the more apparent that man's inhumanity to man will encompass food and drink if we let it.

Take no chances with diet foods while losing weight on the Longevity Diet. Follow the precepts in this chapter and you can have your Longevity and weight loss, too.

THE LIQUID PROTEIN DIET

Another controversial approach to weight loss has been the modified, fast-using liquid protein. A number of deaths among people who were on a liquid protein diet for several months have prompted the Food and Drug Administration to warn the public against using this product on a fasting diet plan without medical advice and supervision.

Because nothing except pure protein is ingested on this plan, the body receives no vitamins and minerals necessary to function properly. You can starve a horse a few days and he will still pull the load. But you can starve him only so long and then he will drop dead.

Nature supplies us with protein in ways that it can be fully used. Meats contain minerals. Animal and plant protein foods contain everything else the body needs.

Potassium is an example. Its absence can lead to heart problems. It is not in liquid protein. A number of people on the liquid protein diet for several months died of heart problems when they had never had symptoms of heart disease before beginning the diet.

Yet, a group of Cleveland physicians have defended the liquid protein as an "enormously successful" product in rapid weight reduction. They point to an average weight loss among 1,300 patients of about 100 pounds in 30 weeks.

The parade of new diet approaches will continue. There will be pills, potions, and packaged products aimed at the 30 million officially obese Americans—30 percent overweight—and the additional estimated 30 million who are overweight but not to that degree. It all adds up to a $10 billion a year industry which, if nothing else, will lighten a lot of wallets and purses.

Ice cream moves to ice milk. Yogurt moves to ice yogurt. All is in the expressed interest of weight reduction, but usually these expressions of interest are in the $10 billion rather than *your* interest.

A quick breakfast food comes out. It is supposed to be nutritious, fast, reasonable, and low in calories. If you want to be adventuresome, buy it. However, if you want to live out your years to the fullest, don't fall for the "pitch." If it is like others on the market, it is just a sweet cookie fortified with fewer nutrients than were removed from the refining of the flour and sugar. And it probably has more calories than the conventional breakfast of juice, milk, and whole grain cereal.

One thing about nature. When it gives you nutrition, it gives and gives and gives. A man-made product has only the nutrients listed on the "fortified" label. Nature throws in many important trace minerals and vitamins we all need.

Now, jubilant researchers are hailing a new diet pill as "the best ever." It's called PPA, short for phenylpropanolamine. I say if you cannot pronounce it, walk carefully.

It causes a mild dryness of the mouth. There are a few reports of slight headaches. Some nausea. Yet, researchers are so convinced that it is the safest of drugs, it is being made available without a prescription.

Are you willing to take a chance?

I'm glad you said "No." The proper nutrition way is the better way. Every time.

You can bet your life.

Chapter 10

Special Diets and Techniques
for Increasing Youthful Energy

Diet was once the major weapon of medicine against health problems. Today, it is largely bypassed by doctors in favor of medicinal approaches.

Food can still be your best medicine, not only preventive medicine but possibly corrective medicine. In these days of higher health care costs, many who delay going to their doctor for every minor complaint might spend that time eating health-giving foods. It might make that trip to the doctor's office unnecessary and give him more time to spend on the seriously ill.

Doctors are in favor of people assuming more responsibility for their own health. In a recent *Readers Digest* article entitled "Doctoring Isn't Just for Doctors,"* Dr. B. Leslie Huffman, Jr., immediate past president of the American Academy of Family Physicians, was quoted as predicting that the increasing involvement of patients in their own health care will be one of the most exciting medical developments in the next ten years.

Pediatricians are teaching mothers to take throat cultures at home when their children are ill. Foot care, diet, stress control,

---

*Condensed from "Medical World News," October 3, 1977.

dental hygiene are just a few of the topics that are being taught by other physicians through community centers and colleges.

To live longer, you need to educate yourself about your body. Take courses. Read books. Follow medical reports simplified in popular magazines and in newspapers.

Don't be your own doctor all the way. Be ready to get help from your family physician. But doctors cannot provide preventive medical care. They are too busy treating problems that have already developed. That is where you come in. Prevent problems. Live longer.

It has been said that the public lacks information and possibly even the good judgment to make decisions on these complex issues of what is good for us and what is not. It has also been admitted that with constant lobbying pressure, the government cannot be relied upon to always make rational judgments.

So you and I must procure more information and make wise decisions.

TO DO OR NOT TO DO— TO EAT IT OR NOT TO EAT IT

Example: Top researchers in Europe and America announce that certain protein-rich foods and certain vitamins can help protect the smoker from toxic cancer-causing gases. The protective ingredients are L-cysteine (an amino acid in protein) and ascorbic acid (vitamin C).

Problem: You are a smoker, what do you do? Does this discovery give you immunity?

Use your own judgment, not mine.

Example: About 25 percent of Americans are lactose intolerant. They have difficulty digesting milk. It can cause abdominal pain, flatulence and other discomfort. It causes an irritable colon syndrome in some people, also ulcerative colitis. An enzyme product becomes available. It comes from yeast. It helps relieve disorders related to lactose intolerance.

Problem: You have trouble with milk. Do you use the new enzyme product and drink more milk?

Again, it is your judgment that counts for you, not my judgment.

Example: A Canadian researcher announces he has slashed the cholesterol content of eggs by 50 percent. He does this by feeding the hens less animal protein and more grain and vegetable compounds called steroids, purported to have no side effects on humans.

Problem: Do you buy the new eggs?

Don't look at me.

Example: You hear that according to a report in the *British Medical Journal*, chest and respiratory illnesses in children are more common in households that use gas for cooking than electricity. A survey of over 5,000 children showed those in homes using gas for cooking had more coughs, chest colds, and bronchitis, believed caused by higher than safe levels of oxides of nitrogen and other products of gas combustion.

Problem: You cook with gas. Your children have respiratory problems. Do you switch to electricity or open the windows?

I'm sorry; I have my own problems.

Example: The Environmental Protection Agency finds that a pesticide used to fumigate Hawaiian pineapple and Florida grapefruit being sent outside the state is hazardous, causing cancer among the workers using it and a lowered male sperm count among the male workers.

Problem: Do you stop eating fresh Hawaiian pineapple and Florida grapefruit until the pesticide (ethylene dibromide) is replaced?

I pose all of these problems to you because they represent the kinds of situations that are continuously arising in our industrialized society.

By the time you read this, these problems may no longer exist, but, I assure you, new ones will have arisen.

If you are ignorant of the existence of these kinds of possible threats to your high level of health, you become just another one of the sheep being led to slaughter.

On the other hand, if you are aware, you might be able to find a hole in the fence.

My own awareness does not necessarily lead me to the same course of action that your awareness might lead you.

I might say that gas provides less of a threat to my respiratory system than the convenience it provides. And because I'm not a pineapple worker, I might say "piffle" to the pesticide risk.

On the other hand, you have every right in the interest of long life to be as cautious as your intuition dictates.

It is a safe rule that unnatural additives to our food or environment are, to a degree, unsafe.

WHAT TO DO ABOUT MINOR COMPLAINTS

When the body whispers that something is not going right, we don't feel right.

When the body speaks softly to remind us, we feel a slight pain or discomfort.

When the body calls out aloud to correct the problem, we hurt.

If we ignore this communication, we could wind up six feet under with an epitaph, "I told you I was sick."

Heed we must. The only problem is when do we seek professional advice?

The delivery of health care to all the people is in crisis. For many, health care, except when the body screams, is not available. Money is one problem, but there are others.

The net result is we usually do not think in terms of going to a doctor when we have a minor discomfort. Still, the body's message cannot be ignored, or that message will get louder.

What do we do?

If your car does not ride properly, you check certain things for which you are responsible. Are the tires inflated? Is there gas in the tank? You need to check whether you have been treating your car properly.

Your body has been depending on you, too. Have you been giving your body what it needs? Here is a maintenance check list that you might use to check your body at the first "whisper" of trouble.

- Have you been eating enough natural protein? (Check against minimum daily protein requirements supplied by each "wonder" food as listed in chapter 3 starting on page 58.)

- Have you been getting enough natural vitamins and minerals?
- Have you been avoiding stress?
- Have you been drinking enough fresh water?
- Have you been getting enough sleep?
- Fresh air?
- Exercise?
- What changes in eating habits have taken place recently, prior to the advent of the discomfort?
- What problems in business life, love life, or social life have arisen about this same time.

The answers to these nine questions might point the finger of suspicion at the cause of your discomfort. It could be dietary or from some other infraction of the physical health rules. Or it could be mental. A stressful event can manifest quite quickly in the physical state.

If we make a correction in the suspected cause and the discomfort disappears, it is safe to say we have hit "pay dirt."

On the other hand, if we make a correction in the suspected cause and the discomfort continues or worsens, the time has come for professional help.

Self-care is on the upswing. More people are watching what they eat. More are jogging. More are playing tennis. Millions have stopped smoking.

As a result, newly-released Census Bureau statistics for the period 1973 to 1975 show fewer heart disease deaths. Four years have been added to the average life expectancy of women and three years have been added for men.

Current life expectancy for all races in the United States is 69 years for men and 76.7 years for women. This varies for different states. Hawaii has the longest, about one year longer than the national average. The District of Columbia is lowest, running some four years below the national average. What price stress?

You can extend your life not only by following the Longevity Diet, but also by being alert to your relationship with your environment and to every signal from your body.

YOU NEED NOT ACCEPT ILLNESS
IN LATER YEARS

The Senior Citizens of today are getting a fast deal from society. Society replies to every complaint, "What do you expect at your age?"

Society considers old age as sexless. Older people are not supposed to enjoy sex. It is for young and middle-aged adults.

Society considers old age as mindless. There is no need to educate older people, and anyhow they don't have the mental capacity to learn.

Society considers old age as an incurable disease. "You might as well accept your condition."

All untrue. Old age is not a creeping death.

Older people enjoy sex on and on.

They take university courses and earn degrees.

They have curative powers to conquer illness.

Recently, a conference on "Changing Images of Aging" was co-sponsored by the Institute for Creative Aging and the University of Southern California. One of the speakers, psychologist Carl Rogers, reported how at the age of 75 he was now more open than ever to new ideas, including psychic research. He said he now feels both pain and joy more intensely than when he was younger.

That does not sound like a person taken over by a creeping death.

At the same conference, Senior Citizen Maggie Kuhn, founder of the Gray Panthers, demanded that the medical profession give up its "accept it at your age" stance. She called for early detection of nutrition problems and stress problems that can lead quickly to nursing homes, and foresaw the formation of wholistic health centers to point the way toward treatment of the body, mind, and spirit.

In the next chapter and also in the final chapter of this book, I am going to give you ways to program yourself free of the necessity to manifest old age in the way society sees it. I just want to say here and now, "Reject old age."

Be just as alert to illness as you can, following the procedures just outlined. Do not accept it as a symptom of old age when illness comes. Assert your right to full recovery. It is always yours.

DIETARY STEPS TO INCREASE PHYSICAL AND SEXUAL ENERGY

One "whispering" of the body is a decrease in energy.

Feelings of not wanting to get up and go places, feelings of exhaustion for no apparent reason, tired feelings when you were never tired under similar circumstances before, feelings of sexual inadequacy or lack of sexual desire—all are communications from your body saying, "All is not as it should be."

Most people can put up with occasional feelings of having reduced energy, but when these feelings infringe on the pleasures of sex, the alarm bell rings.

Then there usually begins a search for a "love" food or aphrodisiac. From the African bush where the hunter chews some bark from the yohimbé tree before going home to his woman, to the tea rooms of China where men sip ginseng brew to restore sexual vitality, there is always a "love" food around.

From the exotic powdered buffalo horn to the common hen's egg, aphrodisiacs have been whispered about and touted. So little scientific investigation has been conducted with any of them, that the reputations of "love" food are usually chalked up to legend.

However, even legends can be therapeutic. The reason is this: The most frequently prescribed "medicine" is not aspirin. It is a sugar pill. You are not told it is a sugar pill. You believe it is medicine that will help you. It does Surely, it is not the sugar. What helps you is the belief that it will help.

This is known as the placebo effect. If somebody raves to you about how chocolate-covered ants restored his sexual vigor instantly, you are "programmed" for this placebo effect.

The greater the reputation, the greater the results.

But before you close your eyes and pop a chocolate-covered ant, I have news for you.

A recent survey of physicians produced a unanimous agreement that the best "love" food is a well-balanced diet high in protein, raw fruits and vegetables. They also agree that excess fat will slow you down in bed and out.

Presumably, you are now on the High Protein Longevity Diet. If not, get on, and your energy level will increase.

However, if you are already on it and still need an energy boost, here are some choices available to you:

THE SHORT FAST AS AN ENERGY BOOSTER

Alternative #1. Go on a one or two-day fast. Eat no solid food. Drink only fruit juice, herb teas, and water. Dr. Alvenia Fulton, a Chicago naturopath who owns a health food store, finds that this is a good way to cleanse the blood system of undigested fats and other accumulations which could be interfering with the proper distribution of nutrients. Drinking plenty of pure water on a fast is a must.

Dick Gregory, social activist and comedian, is an ardent supporter of Dr. Fulton's approach and the father of ten children. He is quoted in *Ebony Magazine* as saying, "If more men knew how fasting affected their sexual behavior, they would be out there drinking Lake Michigan dry."

A fast makes good sense. It gives the body a chance to catch up on its "house cleaning." Most of this catching up is done on the first two days. I am not recommending longer fasts. I am not recommending against them either. Many who have gone on fasts lasting five to ten days have reported great health improvements and a euphoric feeling. Any fast more than two days should be supervised by your physician.

Those first two days are the hardest part of fasting. On the first day, the body's "appestat" calls for fuel and when none comes the hunger pangs scream the body's protest. On the second day, the elimination of poisons is in full swing and the purging process is not pleasant.

When the work is done, the "appestat" is turned down and those who stay on the fast longer than two days report no more symptoms of hunger and misery. It becomes smooth sailing.

However, when you end a two-day fast, your energy level is restored. Your sexual appetite and vigor are heightened. You feel better both physically and mentally.

Lillian S. is 61. She began going on a one-day fast, once a week, fifteen years ago. She has averaged one sick day every two years. Her Longevity Diet tenure goes back even further to thirty years. She looks as if aging stopped in her thirties. She is married, but that does not stop men of all ages, 30 to 70, from admiring her at parties and on the beach.

Drinking plenty of liquids is recommended on your short one or two-day fast. Water is top priority. Next, fruit juices such as apple, orange, and grape.

The only other allowable liquids are herb teas. Camomile tea, made from the flowers, is a soothing brew. Sage tea is said to have a healing effect, its reputation going back to the knights of Chaucer's days who drank sage tea after battle to restore themselves. Mint tea has a refreshing flavor and is soothing to the stomach.

Let tea steep in the boiled water for ten minutes to soak the essence out, then strain. Add lemon or honey, or you may find neither to be necessary.

Fasting can be the answer to your energy crisis. If it is not your cup of tea, there are other alternatives.

THE HIGH PROTEIN, MODIFIED VEGETARIAN DIET FOR SEX POWER

There are two additional approaches to improve sexual and physical energy which are not conflicting and which many have found to be quite compatible. One approach is the vegetarian way. The other proclaims eggs to be the greatest of aphrodisiacs and energy builders.

Alternative #2. Try going on a high protein vegetarian diet for a week or two. Eliminate meat, fish, poultry and dairy products. However, increase your egg intake from the Longevity Diet recommended limit of two whole eggs a week to one or two eggs a day.

Vegetarian sources of protein include soy beans, seeds, and whole grains. Most vegetable proteins are not complete proteins so the vegetarian eats a larger variety in a single meal for best protein absorption. Corn and beans together make a complete protein. Peanut butter and whole grain bread make a complete protein. On the other hand, soy beans alone are complete protein in themselves.

Here are some typical vegetables and their protein content. Also listed are their fat, carbohydrate, and total calories.

Vegetable	Protein Calories	Carbohydrate Calories	Fat Calories	Total Calories
Broccoli (1 cup)	16	—	28	44
Chinese cabbage (1 cup)	4	—	20	24
Carrots, raw (6 tbs.)	4	—	20	24
Celery, two stalks	4	—	8	12
Corn, 1 lg. fresh ear	20	18	120	158
Kale (½ cup)	12	9	28	49
Mustard green (½ cup)	12	—	20	32
Peas, green (¾ cup)	28	—	72	100
Soy beans, fresh (6 tbs.)	131	1	—	132
Spinach, fresh (2 tbs. cooked)	4	—	4	8
Squash, winter (½ cup)	8	—	40	48
Stringbeans, fresh (6 tbs.)	8	—	16	24
Turnips (½ cup)	4	—	16	20
Yam (1 small)	83	—	24	107

Have three or more vegetables each lunch or dinner, favoring soy beans, yams, asparagus, and squash. Eat lots of raw salad with a number of raw vegetables chopped up and added to the lettuce leaves.

Why eggs?

We limit eggs in the Longevity Diet because they are a source of killing cholesterol. However, cholesterol is the base for our sex hormones.

A person who lacks sexual energy may have a temporary need for a hormone boost. Eggs can be the answer.

Eggs go way back as a booster of sexual potency. The ancient literature of the Romans lauds the energy-building quality of eggs. From Kalamazoo to Kenya, men praise eggs today as an aphrodisiac. Many prefer them raw.

If you stay on this High Protein Modified Vegetarian Diet too long, it begins to conflict with the High Protein Longevity Diet. Egg yolks may restore sex hormone levels, but they can also begin to produce excess cholesterol which in turn can begin to cost days off your longer life.

A couple of weeks on the eggs cannot yield a significant increase in cholesterol, especially since you have eliminated altogether animal fat, another cholesterol source.

One man who went on this diet asked me to reinforce its effects with mental instructions at a hypnotic level. Within one week his wife, whose sexual needs were not being met, phoned to ask me to "turn off the power." He was waking up several times during the night and demanding his marital rights.

It is advisable to take two "wonder" foods as vitamin and mineral supplements while on this diet: blackstrap molasses and brewer's yeast. A multi-vitamin product would also be helpful. Lechithin is a substance which helps keep fat from adhering to artery walls. You might consider taking lecithin as a dietary supplement, too.

This brings us to a third alternative.

THE ROLE OF VITAMIN E IN SEXUAL ACTIVITY

There are a number of "wonder" foods and supplements that act as invigorators.

The two just mentioned are top choices. Give these a more frequent position on your daily menus. In fact, make them a daily habit.

Alternative #3. Stay on the Longevity Diet, but make brewer's yeast and blackstrap molasses a daily supplement.

Also add to your daily intake of vitamin E.

Vitamin E's role in sexual activity is not thoroughly understood, but its effects are proven again and again.

Take vitamin E twelve hours apart from blackstrap molasses.

You take the molasses for its iron. But iron destroys vitamin E. Separated in time, they both can go to work for you.

The U. S. Food and Drug Administration, usually reluctant to recognize the importance of vitamins, has conceded that vitamin E represents a clear need in human nutrition.

If the foods identified in Chapter 3 can be called "wonder" foods, then vitamin E is indeed the "wonder" vitamin.

Vitamin E is found in every tissue of the body. Just why is not clear but evidence is pointing to its protective function against incipient destructive oxidation.

Vitamin E is therefore a strong ally of longevity. It is a strong ally of healthful functioning of all organs. It is a strong ally of sexual activity.

The need for vitamin E in animals has been shown to be greater with aging. Vitamin E helps the body to reduce the amount of oxygen locally when a metabolic function might be adversely affected. It is therefore an anti-oxidant.

If cells are not protected against oxidation, they, in effect, burn up. When more cells are destroyed in this manner than are replaced, aging takes place.

The oxidation of fats is increasingly present during aging. Vitamin E is therefore increasingly important for older people.

Vitamin E is non-toxic. It should be taken in its natural, not synthetized form, called tocopherol. It cannot be synthetized by the body.

If you do not provide vitamin E in food or by supplement, the body suffers.

HOW TO INSURE YOU ARE GETTING AN ADEQUATE AMOUNT OF ANTI-AGING VITAMIN E

Although nature supplies us with an abundant supply of vitamin E sources, it is a fragile substance. You may think you are getting your vitamin E but you may be mistaken.

Let us examine the perils that vitamin E must survive in order to arrive at the cells of your body, ready to protect them from aging.

An increased intake of polyunsaturated fatty acids depletes vitamin E. Since the Longevity Diet decreases dangerous saturated fats by replacing them with polyunsaturated fats, an increase in vitamin E is indicated.

Many "wonder" foods contain vitamin E, but you may still want to play it safe by adding vitamin E to your daily mineral and vitamin supplements.

There are some types of vitamin E that are not as biologically active. Beta and gamma tocopherols are less beneficial than alpha tocopherol, the most active vitamin E.

The vitamin E content in food drops sharply with cooking.

For instance, there is vitamin E in corn, but by the time it arrives in front of you in the form of dry (and pre-cooked) flakes, it has only 2 percent of its vitamin E content left.

Just processing corn into white corn meal loses 35 percent of its vitamin E. Wheat loses anywhere from 25 to 90 percent of its vitamin E in processing, rice up to 70 percent.

Besides the processing and cooking of foods as a peril to vitamin E, other foods present can also pose a peril.

I already mentioned iron. It is death to vitamin E. So are fish liver oils. If you eat a food like spinach and a vitamin E food, the vitamin E is cancelled because of the iron in the spinach. Similarly, if you are taking codliver oil as a supplement, it creates a need for additional vitamin E later, to replace what it deactivates. Selenium is a trace metal that is not usually sold at health food stores as it is extremely poisonous. If selenium is part of any mineral supplement prescribed or purchased, do not take vitamin E. The combination can be fatal.

It is alright to eat moderately of foods containing selenium while also taking vitamin E. These foods include wheat germ, brewer's yeast, bran, broccoli, seafood, pork and beef kidney, and Brazil nuts.

Gerontologists Richard J. Passwater and Paul A. Welker of the American Gerontological Research Laboratories report it is their belief that the use of vitamin E, in addition to other anti-oxidants can lengthen the life span in man by five to ten years. In addition, it is their belief that by adding vitamin B complex, vitamin C together with sulfur containing amino acids and other minerals, man's life span can be extended by 30 years of useful life.

It is not speculation. Dr. A. L. Tappel found a 50 percent increase in the life span of mice fed large amounts of vitamin E.

The only thing holding back an explosion of professional enthusiasm for the life-prolonging properties of vitamin E is the scientific understanding of *how* it works. There is no doubt *that* it works.

Make sure you are getting your share of the "Vitamin of Youth"—alpha tocopherol by buying the natural product and taking the capsules once or twice a day after meals. Do not worry about an overdose. It is harmless. But the law of diminishing returns sets in when you are supplying the cells of your body with all they need.

A popular brand of vitamin E might come in strength of 400 international units (I. U.). One or two capsules a day of this strength should make a noticeable difference in your energy and youthful feeling.

Read the fine print. I have a vial in front of me now. It says "400 I. U. d-alpha tocopherol plus added beta, gamma, and delta tocopherols." I look for the "alpha." Alpha is the "muscle" of vitamin E.

WHAT TO DO ABOUT THE SALT PARADOX:
YOU CAN'T LIVE WITH IT OR WITHOUT IT

Sodium and chlorine are two elements that are essential to the body. Combined they form salt—sodium chloride.

You see it on every table where people eat. "It makes food taste better" is the accepted reason.

Actually, the real reason is that the body requires salt. The kind we put on the table though is good only in an emergency. The body can use salt tablets in a heat spell to replace the salt leeched out of our body by excessive perspiration. But as a daily fare, the body prefers organic salt, the kind of sodium chloride that is part of plant material. It can readily absorb vegetable salt but it can use only a limited amount of inorganic or table salt.

This ordinary white table salt belongs in the same family as ordinary white sugar and ordinary white flour. It is foreign to the body and poses more problems to the body than it solves.

Take a look into your neighbor's kitchen. Mrs. Jones is at the kitchen range now. She has already added salt three times to the stew. Now she is salting the vegetables. I don't believe it: She is salting the garlic bread before toasting it.

What Mrs. Jones does not realize is that the common table salt put on food being cooked hardens the grain. Starch especially becomes harder to digest if cooked with salt.

Not only that, but the body treats common table salt as an unwanted product. The kidneys must excrete it. If the kidneys are not healthy enough to do the job, the salt remains in the blood. Some is deposited in the tissues and some clogs tiny arteries.

The many mineral salts that are in water are thought by many natural health authorities to be the major cause of senility and stroke.

What then is the answer? It is: Use organic salt—the kind your body can use to its advantage. Vegetable salt is available in health food stores. It usually comes iodized, that is iodine has been added because it has been largely removed from the soil through generations of cultivation and not replaced.

The Longevity Diet should provide enough sodium chloride for your body's needs. Relatively high levels of sodium are found in meat, fish, poultry, milk and milk products. It is also found in celery, spinach, kale, chard, carrots, beets and other vegetables.

However, your taste buds may have become hypnotized by salt, like they have been by those other two white unmentionables. If so, the iodized vegetable salt should replace the common table salt, for uncommonly good health.

It is up to you.

You can choose to smoke. If so, there is little that a doctor can do for a lung that is blackened and overinflated by smoking.

You can choose to drink heavily. If so, there is little that a doctor can do about a liver that is progressively de-activated.

You can choose to worry and tense up in stressful situations. If so, there is little that a doctor can do about your continuing stomach ulcers and the complications they can eventually cause.

You can choose salt and pepper, sugar and flour, and all the wrong starchy and fatty, quick and easy foods. If so, there is little that a doctor can do about your life expectancy.

What I am really saying is that longevity is largely a matter of choice.

What's yours?

Chapter 11

Protecting Yourself from Health Enemy No. 2—Stress

If food—too much or the wrong kind—can be the number one cause of our physical demise, then health enemy number two can be none other than stress.

Stress is a newcomer to the health menaces. People have been overstuffing or undernourishing their bodies from the beginning of time. But it has taken modern civilization to provide the kind of stress that kills.

There is a place on earth where heart attacks are almost unknown. It is 12,000 feet high in the Peruvian Andes. There has been only one fatal heart attack in the past decade among the 72,000 Peruvian Indians.

Doctors who have studied these people agree that there are three factors that contribute to this incredible situation:

1. Altitude
2. No-fat diet
3. Life style

When people live at high altitudes in oxygen-thin air, the body must compensate to meet its oxygen requirements. This brings about a strengthening of the cardiovascular system,—better arteries, stronger hearts.

The stronger hearts of the Peruvian Indians are not pounded by our two greatest health enemies. The people eat hardly any fat. Vegetables and potatoes comprise some 90 percent of their diets. No fat means no excess cholesterol lining the arteries and causing the heart to have to pump harder to get the blood circulating.

Also, they have an easy going life style. They get up when the sun rises. They work only if they wish to. They wish to work only when there is a need to plant some vegetables or pick them. They have no schedule. They eat when the sun is high in the sky. They go to sleep when they are tired.

When the Peruvian Andes dweller leaves the high altitudes and migrates down towards the sea, the air gets thinner, the food gets fattier, his life gets busier and he becomes susceptible to heart disease.

Some 50 percent of our deaths in the United States are due to cardiovascular causes. Even if we could figure out how to live in thin air, we could not strengthen our hearts and arteries against the enemies *fat* and *stress*. Even the Peruvian Indian with his stronger system succumbs to them when he descends to "where the action is."

But we can control fat if we know how, and presumably you now know how. And we can control stress.

In this chapter we will learn how to tame this killer.

WORRY, FEAR AND ANXIETY: WEAPONS OF STRESS

Bob Hope eats no fried food. He has stopped drinking and smoking. He enjoys only decaffeinated coffee and watches his diet. As you know, he is fit and active at 75.

But the real secret to the famous comedian's youthful looks and energy is the fun he derives in entertaining. He laughs and is able to make others laugh.

If you are laughing and having fun, you cannot be worrying or fearing, and you cannot be anxious and concerned. Worry, fear, anxiety, and chronic concern are the tools or weapons of stress.

Laughter is a great weapon against stress, but there are other weapons. We cannot all be comedians. But we can be in control of stress.

Some people are under intense stress only under special conditions. They may feel stress at high places or in an elevator or in an airplane. These stresses are due to phobias usually related to some past experience. There are techniques to trace these back to their sources and then to dispel them through understanding.

The main thrust of this chapter will not be on these special causes of stress known as phobias, but rather on the chronic causes of stress which we cannot escape by turning on the lights or leaving a small room.

The real threats to longevity are the kinds of stress that we do not seem to be able to escape from,—the stress we feel from other people with whom we live or work; the stress we feel about not enough money coming in and too much going out; the stress we feel from the need to compete, advance, and succeed.

People compete, advance, and succeed every day with a minimum of stress. What do they have that a person who experiences maximum stress does not have? The answer is self-confidence.

Self-confidence is never misplaced.

That sounds like a pretty bold statement. It reminds one of the joke about the psychiatrist who, after months of analysis, tells the patient, "You have an inferiority complex because you are really inferior."

Self-confidence is never misplaced because the person who has it creates in himself the very person in which he is confident.

The opposite is true, too. Lack of self-confidence creates a person not deserving of confidence.

Anthony C., a commercial photographer, was terrified every time he got a call from an advertising agency to "shoot" on a project. He would be bathed in perspiration before he hung up the phone. He felt like doubling over to form a fetus and crawling back into the womb.

When he arrived on the set, he was rigid with fear. Would he succeed? "I was always afraid they would reject my work. I remembered when I was a child and the boys would not let me play softball with them. They called me stinky." Would he get paid? Or would they call him stinky?

Anthony was beginning to get chronic stiff necks, headaches, and other physical "miseries." His nerves were shot. He was always tense. He had feelings of despair about his career.

When he came to me, it was to help him with his traumatic fear of failure. I taught him Hypno-Cybernetics*, a simple way to relax and turn confidence-lack into abundance.

In a few weeks, Anthony was enjoying life like never before. "I can enjoy Saturday and Sunday," he said, "without fear of Monday and Tuesday." He went from fear and trepidation about his work to eagerness and excitement. As his self-confidence improved, his photographs improved, confirming the validity of his self-confidence and reinforcing it.

If you were tense and I were to say to you, "Relax," you would very likely tense up more. You might even snap back at me, "I *am* relaxed!"

Telling somebody to relax is not helping that person. Providing a method to relax is quite a different, more constructive approach. I am going to give you several methods to relax. I am sure you are going to enjoy them.

Why relax? When you are relaxed, you are able to change habitual ways of thinking that are interfering with your effectiveness as a person.

Through relaxation, you can give your own mind instructions that your mind will accept—instructions to combat anxieties, worries, and other causes of stress.

HOW TO RELAX AND RIDE ROUGHSHOD OVER STRESSFUL CONDITIONS

You cannot relax while you are reading this book. Your body might be relaxed, but your mind is active.

So, to experience the methods of relaxation I am now going to give you, you need to put the book down and do it, just as you have to put the book down to carry out recipe instructions.

For instance, if I were to ask you to close your eyes and take a deep breath. Then imagine yourself surrounded by a gray cloud

---

*"Hypno-Cybernetics: Helping Yourself to a Rich New Life," Petrie and Stone, Parker Publishing Co., Inc., 1973.

and getting heavier in the chair, you would have to stop reading to experience that.

Why not read the above paragraph again, then put the book down and do it, telling yourself as you end your relaxation that you will feel better than before. Count to three and open your eyes.

I'll wait. . . . .

Good. I'm sure you do feel better. However, the best is yet to come. After you have practiced this a few times and been able to deepen your relaxation, you will be ready to use simple "instructions" to your mind that will insulate you from stress.

Insulation from stress can contribute as much to your longevity as cutting fat intake in half.

After you practice the above simple relaxation, you might like to try a more complete relaxation session. I will give you the text for one now. It cannot be read while you relax, so you might get somebody to read it slowly to you. Or you might want to tape it and then play it back, so that your own calm, quiet voice will be speaking slowly to you.

I am very comfortable . . . I am sitting loosely, limply in the chair . . . my feet are flat on the floor . . . my hands are on my lap or hanging down . . . I am very comfortable.

I am looking at the ceiling now . . . at a fixed point . . . I am staring at the ceiling . . . all my attention is focused at the fixed point on the ceiling. My eyelids are getting tired from looking at the point on the ceiling. I am very comfortable. I am taking a slow deep breath and exhaling very slowly . . . I am becoming aware of a very comfortable feeling with each breath I take. I am taking another deep breath—I hold it while I count to five and then let it out slowly. One . . . two . . . three . . . four . . . five. I enjoy that nice, pleasant, comfortable sensation in my abdomen. As I relax there comes a feeling of heaviness. I feel this heaviness and now I am relaxed.

My eyes are still occupied with the point I have selected on the ceiling. I am becoming aware of my feet . . . the soles of my feet are more relaxed . . . they are becoming heavier and heavier. My feet are becoming heavier . . . moment by moment . . . heavier and heavier. The heaviness creeps up into my ankles . . . the feet and ankles . . . heavier and heavier . . . up the legs into the thighs.

My whole body feels heavier and heavier. It is so pleasant and comfortable. The heaviness creeps into the chest . . . up the hands and arms into the neck. Now my whole body from the neck down feels heavy . . . the feet . . . the ankles . . . the legs . . . the thighs . . . the abdomen . . . the chest—heavy—heavy—heavier. My jaws begin to relax . . . the lower jaw relaxes and now my mouth opens slightly . . . My jaws are limp and loose . . . teeth apart . . . lips apart. I am so relaxed my eyelids begin to blink. I will let them blink . . . I will not fight to keep my eyes open . . . I will let them close. I will keep them closed. I will not fight to keep them open . . . I will relax completely . . . I will close them now . . . I will close them and keep them closed.

With my eyes closed . . . I can visualize a darkness—the color grey or black. My mind is empty of thoughts. I am thinking of nothing . . . I am doing nothing. That's the secret of relaxation. I will relax all over now—in my mind and in my body . . . just relax and enjoy the nice comfortable feeling. I will breathe slowly and deeply, exactly as if I were asleep—and with each breath . . . I go deeper . . . deeper and deeper into relaxation . . . deeper and deeper relaxed . . . soon I will be as close to sleep as it's possible to get and yet remain conscious and cooperative. So comfortable . . . breathing slowly and deeply and enjoying every moment.

It's a pleasant sensation and I know that even in the deepest stage of relaxation, I am no more unconscious than I am now. There will always be an awareness. It's a kind of detached feeling . . . I can ignore what I wish to ignore and pay attention only to what I need and want to pay attention to.

I keep right on relaxing—going deeper and deeper. I am learning to understand with my unconscious mind and I am learning to understand with my conscious mind. I am learning from this experience. I am learning more about myself. I see myself as more competent. The more capable I see myself, the more capable I become . . . I have confidence in myself, more and more with each passing hour. I can learn by myself through my own efforts. Now I want time to seem infinitely long, infinitely l-o-n-g and then slowly and gradually I will arouse myself slowly and gradually awake . . . arousing . . . arousing . . . knowing I can go back again some other time. Arousing . . . arousing . . . and now all of me has awakened and I feel fine . . . now I am wide awake. I will move or twist around in the chair and reorient myself.

THE BRAIN AS A SERVOMECHANISM

There are many relaxation tapes now available. They are all good. They all help you to relax. But the above relaxation is better. There is a subtle reason.

The tape that helps you relax might be compared to taking an aspirin when you have a bacterial infection.

The relaxation I have given you, whether read to you by another person or taped with your own voice, might be compared to an aspirin plus an antibiotic to fight the infection.

The antibiotic in the above relaxation is the statement about learning more about yourself and becoming more capable and confident.

This is the part that fights the cause of the stress.

If you are tense and you listen to a relaxation tape that does not get at the cause of the tenseness—this is usually lack of self-confidence in your ability to cope—then you are giving your brain two sets of opposite instructions.

One set is the "no confidence" instructions which pushed the alarm button to begin with that started the stress.

The second set is "relax, ignore stress."

These two sets of instructions are opposite. Fed into a computer, it could not compute.

Your brain is such a computer. It is a servomechanism programmed to behave you.

Give it conflicting instructions and you produce conflict. Conflict produces more stress.

So, you need to get to the cause of the stress.

Self-criticism is a downer. It undermines self-confidence. The next situation that arises which requires your participation activates that lack of confidence. Result: stress.

So you need to give your servomechanism new programming. You need to affirm your trust in yourself.

This, too, can cause a conflict. If you are convinced you are a "nogoodnik," telling yourself you are a superstar will be like spinning your wheels. You will get nowhere. "Does not compute," will be the reply from your confused servomechanism. More stress.

Can you remember when you did a job right? Can you recall when you did something correctly. Of course you can. You can remember hundreds. I ask you now to make a list. This list might include:

- Poured over 1,000 cups of tea and coffee without spilling a drop.
- Found my way from here to there hundreds of times without error.
- Made scores of new friends.
- Wrote dozens of correct letters.
- Made it on time to countless appointments.

If you are in business, your list might also include the times you closed a successful deal, made a good sale, or conducted a profitable project.

If you are a student, your list might include the good marks you got on certain tests and the times you proved yourself scholastically in other ways.

Whatever your life style, you have reason after reason to be proud of yourself. Instead, you dwell on the failures, the embarrassments, the mistakes.

This list will change the polarity of your self-thoughts from negative to positive.

You will need this list to proceed with the next stress-combating step, so, again, I'll wait . . .

Here is what I want you to do with the list:

1. Sit in a comfortable chair.
2. Do the first (abbreviated short form) relaxation given you on page 199.
3. Open your eyes, look at the list, and daydream about events on the list. Relive them. Be aware of the feelings of self-value that come to you, as you do this.
4. End by affirming, "I am competent and capable."

It will do you absolutely no good to read these four steps. You need to experience them. Experiencing is programming your servomechanism.

Yes, you are programming it to be more confident in yourself. But this diminishes stress. Stress kills.

So you are programming yourself to live longer.

CONQUERING NEGATIVE ATTITUDES
THAT ERODE HEALTH

Stress **is** the big killer. But we harbor many emotional killers within our personalities which also harm us. Many of them in turn cause stress, as we discussed about lack of self-confidence.

The attitudes that are most obviously stress-oriented are:

Anger	Retaliation	Confusion
Hate	Indignation	Indecision
Frustration	Suicidal	Insecurity

Although not obviously so, these attitudes are also stress-oriented:

Remorse	Dejection	Discouragement
Bitterness	Resentment	Depression
Jealousy	Disillusionment	Indignation

You can turn any one of these negative health-eroding attitudes into their positive counterparts using the same method you used for self-confidence, capability, and competency.

Here are the steps:

1. Relax.
2. Daydream about the negative attitude.
3. Make mental affirmations that you are acquiring the positive counterpart of that attitude.

You can relax with the "short form" or "long form" that I have given you.

When you daydream about, say, resentment—ask yourself some questions. When was the last time you were resentful? Why? Was it valid? Was it worth taking years off your life? Can you resolve it philosophically?

When you can answer yes to this last question, you are ready to go "positive." You affirm mentally, "I am no longer resentful. Instead, I feel compassion and understanding."

You know the positive counterparts. For anger it is serenity; for hate it is love. The opposite of frustration is satisfaction. The opposite of retaliation is reconciliation; indignation—charity; suicidal—survival; confusion—calmness; indecision—decisiveness; insecurity—confidence; remorse—forgiveness; bitterness—benevolence; jealousy and envy—forbearance and magnanimity; dejection—enthusiasm; disillusionment—optimism; discouragement—hope and encouragement; depression—elation; and indignation—charity.

It will do little good to take the fats, starches, excessive calories and poisons out of your diet, if you continue to pollute your mind with poisonous attitudes and thoughts. I don't want it said of my Longevity Diet what is sarcastically said of some surgical operations: It was a success but the person died.

Actually, the Longevity Diet is protection against yourself. Natural aging is accelerated by worry, anxiety, fear, and other stress-producing attitudes and emotions.

Nutrition factor minus stress factor = longevity.

That is an oversimplified formula for survival. There are other causal factors, like weather conditions, heredity, etc. But these are the two that are most controlling. Fortunately, they are also the two that you are most in control of.

DAYDREAMING FOR HEALTH

A study of relaxation was conducted recently at the Temple University School of Dentistry. Using biofeedback devices that measure brain waves, skin galvanic resistance, muscle activity, pulse and blood pressure—all indicators of mental and physical relaxation—a team of researchers discovered that simple daydreaming brought about the same depth of relaxation as such advanced techniques as hypnosis and meditation.

Just thinking pleasant thoughts can be just as good for your health as the relaxation that comes with more sophisticated methodology. Here is what happens when you think about beautiful places, pleasant people, doing what you like to do, and other joyful scenes. You turn off stress. You cease being on guard as you continually are in business, social or professional life. You let go of the facade that you create for people around you. You stop playing a role. You become yourself. You are free momentarily of the apprehension and the tension. You let go physically and mentally.

This is the very definition of relaxation. It is stress dissolving.

Daydream.

Daydream about beautiful spots you have visited. Daydream about being with people you enjoy. Daydream about that trip you took or that picnic you went on. Daydream about happy times.

Take a few minutes at the office to "goof off." Close your eyes and daydream.

Some daydreams take an unusual turn. They turn out to be creative. Relaxing to daydream permits problem-solving thoughts to enter your mind.

It's like when you try to remember a name. It does not come. But then when you stop trying, it later pops into your mind.

A busy mind is a tense mind. That tenseness keeps out creative thoughts. As soon as you let go of your tenseness by giving up the struggle for a moment to daydream, solutions have a chance to pop in.

Let them be an extra bonus for your daydreaming. But let the real prize be a few extra months or years at the end of the line.

HOW TO KEEP YOUR JOB FROM KILLING YOU

"I'm just a mechanic," replied Charles McD. when I suggested his migraine headaches might be due to job stress. "I'm no executive with important problems."

I drew him out more about his job. He had quotas to fill and deadlines to meet. He was racing the clock all day and fighting to keep costs down.

Charles half-heartedly agreed to learn to relax and give himself mental instructions like, "There is always time for what I need to do. The more I do, the easier doing becomes, and the more I can do with no sweat."

That was the end of the migraine headaches. It was not at the expense of productivity. Quite the opposite. Charles was able to produce more in his less "up tight" state and he could do so free of pain.

Contrary to what most people believe, job stress has been found to be greater at the bottom of the occupational ladder than it is at the administrative top. A federal study of over 20,000 people in Tennessee in over 100 different occupations discovered that the most harmful stress occurs among factory workers and building laborers. Secretaries and typists, laboratory and dentist technicians, and assembly line workers—all suffered the greatest stress.

Even people in limited supervisory jobs, the so-called middle managers, suffered more stress than top executives. Even nurses suffered more stress than doctors.

The study was conducted by a team from the National Institute for Occupational Safety and Health. It reviewed death certificates and health records at hospitals, and it made on-the-spot inspections of working and psychological conditions.

One of the greatest incidences of stress came among workers who were paid on an incentive basis rather than hourly and where a machine or assembly line dictated the pace of the worker.

Even if you are a top executive with no worry about bills, with several vacations a year, and with a chance to take time off to play golf, you still have stress. The profit motive is constant stress. Holding one's place in the firm or the firm's place in the industry, is stress.

Insulate yourself from stress, regardless of where you are on the job ladder. Use relaxation and positive instructions to yourself. Be able to do this anywhere, anytime—at the drop of a routine.

Stand at the water cooler and close your eyes as you sip the water. Take a deep breath. Envelope yourself in a gray cloud that blocks out the company. Tell yourself, "I am serene. I am in control. I am efficient. I am relaxed." Open your eyes. Take a final sip and you have released any stress that may have been creeping up on you, while at the same time insulating yourself (for awhile) against more stress.

Do this again in the lavatory, at a coffee break, during lunch hour, after work.

Consider stress as a constant menace, waiting to do its dirty work.

STRESS AT HOME AND HOW TO HANDLE IT

Anger lurks in every family. It is the chief domestic source of stress. Spouse angers at spouse, child at parent, parent at child.

Other sources of stress exist, too. The housewife who feels pressured by time is under constant stress.

Virginia K. never had time enough. She scrubbed, she washed, she dusted, she polished and there was always more to do and no time left in the day to do it. She had frequent headaches and came to me for relaxation and mental conditioning. Obviously, I had to find out why Virginia needed to keep her house so sparkling clean.

It took hypnosis ultimately to find the answer. When Virginia was a child, her friend across the street died from blood poisoning. Virginia's parents had warned Virginia she must keep herself clean or if she cut herself, she, too, would get an infection and die.

Today, Virginia was the victim of fear of dirt. Her phobia was causing constant stress and if not dispelled could cause serious health problems, a lot more serious than an infected cut.

Virginia was taught how to relax and while relaxed was given new information about the body's ability to cope with germs. Gradually, she became less anxious about keeping everything in her house sterile. The headaches went away. She began to have time and energy to spare to enjoy life.

Life enjoyed is a longer life than life endured under stress.

Getting back to anger, its harm comes whether the anger is expressed or not. Fits of temper, knockdown drag-out shouting arguments, violent outbursts—all these create acute strain. This is sudden physical stress on the heart and other organs.

But repressed anger—anger felt but not expressed—can be even more insidious. It smoulders within, lasts longer, and consumes cell life.

The 1977 World Congress of Psychiatry in Hawaii received international publicity for its denunciation of Soviet uses of psychiatric tools against dissenters. But an important finding by a panel of six top psychiatrists received little notice. As Dr. Samuel Silverman, Associate Clinical Professor of Psychiatry at Harvard

University put it, "Unexpressed anger is an emotional killer." He said that repressed rage can cause an internal conflict which is often followed by disease. A person who learns how to overcome this can live as much as 15 years longer.

Loneliness is another stressful factor in the home which takes its place alongside of repressed anger as a killer. Older people confined in institutions and cut off from loved ones, age more rapidly. Even dogs are known to die when removed from their masters.

The panel of psychiatrists noted that in the regions of the country where people survive to 100 and more, if a spouse dies, a person will find a new companion, usually within six months.

It was pointed out that many lonely or angry people tend to drink too much. They can then develop cirrhosis of the liver. I know lonely and angry people who tend to overeat. Either way, it is like jumping out of the frying pan into the fire.

Loneliness strikes frequently during holidays. Many people are susceptible to the holiday blues but people who live alone who once knew a family life are likely to be hit hardest by holiday stress.

Symptoms show up before Thanksgiving because it is traditionally family-centered. Then Christmas and New Year's Eve can be an emotional "wipe-out."

Holidays are a time to be happy. If you are not happy, that fact becomes magnified during holidays. As a result, even people in a close family situation experience more stress during holiday seasons.

Mother cooks all day for the holiday dinners and realizes even more dramatically how thankless her family is. Dad works harder and romanticizes the events only to find the nerves of his family taut and irritation rampant. Children vie against each other for parental affection and grow tense as Christmas gifting approaches.

Knowing about these holiday sources of stress can lead to obvious ways to head them off. If you are alone, attend the local mayor's Thanksgiving dinner, even though you deplore receiving handouts. The company is the real gift that the mayor is handing out. Seek company on holidays wherever you can find it. Dull company is better than the cutting stress of loneliness. If a family person, you need to become a family statesman, philosopher and peace maker during stressful holidays.

To live those extra 15 years, free of suppressed anger and loneliness, you need to make decisions and carry them out.

You need to decide that you will think about anger once in awhile before anger-causing situations arise: Why do you get angry? Is it ego? Is it immaturity? What is it? Then you need to think a second time about anger when the impulse to become angry strikes: Is it worth it? What good does it do? What bad does it do?

In other words, think twice before getting angry. You will find that anger is less an impulsive characteristic of the personality and that, rather, the choice is yours.

If you have total confidence in yourself, then you love yourself more, and you can love and understand others. When you can have this understanding rapport with others, you can dismiss anger just by making a decision to do it.

Loneliness can be handled the same way. You need to make a decision that you will be patient until the right person comes along or until temporary separations from loved ones end. You need to keep busy and to be with groups of people whenever possible.

This is a big subject. It cannot be handled with step-by-step instructions in a few pages. My book, *Hypno-Cybernetics* goes ito the problem of handling stress in your life with detailed ways to relax and to program your brain to respond positively to life's stresses.

If I had to sum up into one umbrella statement how to free yourself of the killing effects of stress, I would say, "Get fun out of life." If you are having fun, you are free of stress.

Acquire a philosophy of "live and let live." Live life as if it were a fun game.

Life's conditions are stressful because of the way *you* react to them. You can roll with life's punches. That's fine. But there is a better way. See each condition not as a punch, but as a push, helping you to better and better days.

And more of them.

Chapter 12

Protecting Yourself from Other Health Enemies

The DNA molecule maintains "headquarters" in the nucleus of every cell of our bodies. This DNA is millions of years old, yet shows no signs of aging. It appears to renew itself in the mother's egg and father's sperm. These combine to form a new individual who then carries on the unbroken chain of human life and, in the process, the immortality of the DNA.

So the DNA seems to use us to keep itself going. Individuals are discarded like a snake shedding skin after skin, with the DNA continuing generation after generation.

Theoretically, if we could stop doing whatever warrants our being shed, we could live as long as the DNA molecule.

We are doing plenty that needs to stop. What we know about that we need to stop doing has been discussed up until now. Undoubtedly, there is much more that we do not know.

We are also not doing plenty that we need to start to do. Little things and big things not done can cost us degrees of health. We cannot afford one degree if we are to keep up with the DNA.

Little things we are not doing can fill a book. For instance, even if you are eating raw fruit every day, you may be permitting it to ripen in ways that lose the peak of its nutritional value. Left in a bag, in the refrigerator, or open in a bowl, the unripe fruit seems to go from unripe to rotten, with no time of nutritional ripeness in between.

We are not ripening fruit correctly.

Most fruit is picked green but mature. This means it can be shipped to market without excessive bruising and still complete the ripening process en route. When it arrives in our homes, it is not always fully ripe. We keep it in a bag, maybe unrefrigerated. One day it is not ripe, and the next day one side is ripe while the other side becomes shriveled and overripe.

Recently, scientists of the University of California at Davis, in cooperation with the California Tree Fruit Agreement* growers, developed a ripening bowl. Although specifically designed for California summer fruits, the bowl is applicable to the storage of most unripe fruit.

It is a transparent plastic bowl with a cover to match. Both bowl and cover have venting holes. These holes together with the venting holes around the perimeter are designed to drain off heavier than air carbon dioxide and to allow enough air movement to prevent excess water vapor from collecting. Carbon dioxide and water vapor are produced by fruit ripening.

Also produced by the ripening fruit is an odorless gas called ethylene which induces and promotes the ripening process. The design of the bowl maintains proper levels of ethylene to promote ripening.

So the bowl provides an ideal climate for fast, uniform ripening of fresh peaches, plums, nectarines, pears and many other fruits. It is kept on a dining room table where the fruit can be seen, checked for ripeness and used as a snack or dessert. When all the fruit placed in the bowl is only partially ripe, one or two ripe bananas or other ripe fruit should be added to assist the ripening process.

A ripe fruit usually has even color and is slightly soft to the touch.

A small thing maybe, but properly ripened fruit is worth more to the cells of your body.

---

*California Tree Fruit Agreement, P. O. Box 255383, Sacramento, California 95825.

There may be other small things covered in this chapter from time to time. They will be interspersed with the big "sins of omission"—things we are not doing, that need to be done in the interests of longevity.

MOTION AS A PROTECTIVE TONIC TO THE BODY

Muscles do a lot of tasks inside of our body. They suck in air through our lungs, push food through our intestinal tract, regulate blood pressure, beat our heart, and hold our organs in place.

A muscle weakens if not fully used. Muscles gently challenged respond by becoming better muscles. As the late Paul Bragg used to say, "To rest is to rust."

Don't think I am about to climb aboard the "daily dozen" band wagon. Setting up exercises and I are not on talking terms.

But I do deplore the sedentary life that modern appliances and machines permit. Many of us hardly walk any more. We ride cars and buses and trains. We do not climb anymore; we use elevators. We are no longer sports participants. We are lounge-chair sports spectators.

Muscles are neglected. Stomachs sag. Internal organs are displaced and their functioning becomes less efficient.

The heart is really a muscle. It, too, responds to challenge and becomes a better heart.

The scene is a marathon race. There are hundreds of participants for the Sunday run of 26 miles. Fifty of the participants wear a jersey with a special emblem on it. It is a red heart with a crack in it. These are cardiac patients. They are running for their lives.

These fifty are in a Honolulu Cardiac Rehabilitation Program headed by Dr. Jack H. Scaff, Jr. It recognizes the need for an exercise program as an alternative need for people with coronary disease.

When the program began in 1973, the insurance company for the program predicted five deaths a year, basing that figure largely on the fact this is what would be normal for a group of heart patients. Now, four and one-half years later, among the participants under 70 who are non-smokers, there have been no heart attacks and no deaths.

The heart is a muscle. When you flex a muscle, you strengthen it. It used to be accepted belief that exercise was not good for you unless you had been exercising all of your life. But now programs have been conducted, like at Laguna Hills, California, which show that physical exercise can have beneficial effects when undertaken at any age, even well up into the seventies and eighties.

Like diet, the sooner you start with exercise, the more preventive of disease it is. Also like diet, any change you undertake in your physical activity should be done under the supervision of your physician.

Of course, I am not recommending that you participate in 26-mile marathons. I am recommending that you move about more. Calisthenics are unnatural. They are substitutes for the real thing. The real thing is walking, moving, climbing, working.

The mental attitude is part of the therapy. Calisthenics invite a get-it-over-with attitude. It is drudgery. It is a man-made routine.

Nature's way is more therapeutic because it is fun and exhilerating. Would you rather look at the worn-out carpet while doing push-ups or at the green grass and distant hills while taking a brisk walk. The relaxed mind is a partner to health.

Mild forms of exercise have been found to assist chronically depressed people. The average person feels a sense of relaxation from tension after a 15-minute walk. Here are some of the mild forms of exercise that you might consider adding to your daily life:

- Take early morning brisk walks.
- Take evening strolls.
- Jog a few minutes.
- Climb a few flights of stairs instead of taking the elevator.
- Do some fixing-up around the house.
- Create a balcony, porch, or lanai garden.
- Cut grass or do gardening.
- Play a backyard, park or beach game.

When you exert yourself physically, the heart beats faster to pump more blood through the cell feeding system. Tiny capillaries that have been starved because of poor circulation now get a surge of life-giving oxygen. You feel tingly and exhilerated.

Less of you is dying.

MOVEMENTS THAT MAKE YOU MORE ALERT

The tiny capillaries that receive a surge of life-giving blood when the body moves include those in the brain.

A sedentary life invites earlier senility. Senility is the partial inactivation of brain cells due to starvation. Tiny capillaries become permanently blocked. There is only partial memory, partial logic, partial thinking process.

Movements of the body that cause the heart to beat a little faster help. But any movements help. They keep tissues flexible. They assist bodily fluids to reach every cell. They challenge and build.

Non-strenuous movements should not replace strenuous movements. They should replace no movements. When you are sitting, standing, or waiting, think of some movement you can do.

Waiting for a bus? Don't just look to the left. Make a circular motion with your head. Start by looking down at your feet. Then roll your head to the left, around to the back so you are looking up, then to the right and down again. Do this three times, then three times in the opposite direction.

If other people look at you strangely, explain how it helps circulation to the head and makes you all the more alert in the office. If the bus driver arrives and finds the whole group doing it, don't explain. It may interfere with his driving.

Stretching is healthy movement. Watch the way a cat or a dog does it. Formalize your stretching in the morning when you get out of bed. Stretch your whole body. Start with your arms, then your legs, then put yourself on a make-believe torture rack that stretches you from head to foot, but you'll find it ecstacy not torture.

During the day, take off your footwear while at the desk. Wiggle your toes, rotate your ankles. Move your shoulders in a rotary manner. Take three deep breaths to expand your lungs.

There is no intent in these suggestions to tell you specific things to do. Anything you do is good. Motion is good for the body. It helps maintain youth.

Motion is good for the brain. It helps to keep your brains thirty billion neurons electrified and sparking.

Also, there is safety in motion, as opposed to taking on new exercises or more strenuous forms of sports or activities.

For example, a person can become carried away with jogging. The challenge of jogging just a little further may exceed the physical stress limit of some weak link in the body's chain of organs. Deaths have occurred among persons who are jogging. There will undoubtedly be more. It does not mean that jogging a few minutes is dangerous. It means we do not know our own limits. Anything done to excess is harmful.

Who was it that said even moderation carried to extreme is excess?

But I disagree with the professional school that says that limits of longevity are set by heredity, and that we either cut down on it with smoking, poor nutrition, etc., or maximize it with healthful habits.

A professional trainer of athletics used weights to challenge muscles. His gym was a mass of bars and pulleys. Each day a football player would work with added weight that the muscles were asked to move. Weighted shoes were used in running—more and more weights to challenge the body.

He, himself, used his own equipment. He, too, jogged with increasingly weighted shoes. One day he dropped dead jogging at the age of 62. In most people's eyes, this was a defeat of his concept. But what they did not know was, this man's father and his father before him as far back as the family could remember had died before the age of 55. He had succeeded in breaking his "inherited" limit of longevity.

You do not have to use physical force to break inherited life expectancy tendencies. All you need to do is observe natural life-giving nutrition and stress-avoiding tactics. You will live longer than your forefathers because you will be changing inherited and learned mental and nutritional behavior.

The sins of our fathers are paid for. We need only to pay for our own sins—sins of commission and sins of omission.

Motion and exercise are "food" to our bodies. You can end this sin of omission today. Move!

HOW BODY MOTION RELIEVES STRESS AND
BRINGS OTHER SIDE DIVIDENDS

In examining negative features of today's society, sociologists are able to identify the need for motion to relieve stress.

They see in the labor strike at least a partial cause to be: relief from boredom. There is more excitement in a strike meeting and in picketing than in the monotony of production line work. They recommend not only a tea or coffee break but a stress break for employees to exercise, play ping pong and enjoy other activities together that adjust levels of stress.

They see in hooliganism, vandalism and other crimes of violence, the need to release tension and stress. Youngsters especially need to work off physical energy and generate adrenalin and other body fluids in the process.

Activities that involve body motion not only provide support for body life-support systems but provide a safety valve to let off "steam,"—steam that is the cause of nervous tension and mental stress.

We have already discussed stress. It is a deadly weapon. It is wielded by life itself. We need to live life in a way that minimizes our exposure to that weapon and to release ourselves from its effects as frequently as possible.

Mental and physical relaxation procedures provided in the previous chapter are preventive. Physical activity of an enjoyable nature is therapeutic.

Its therapy derives not only from the relief of stress, but from other effects as well, depending on the nature of the activity.

A man I knew once built a boat in his back yard. He knew nothing about building boats, but when that boat was placed in the water, that man was "ten feet tall." His job was non-creative, boring. Building a boat gave him a sense of accomplishment that many a psyche needs in order to have the will to live.

Yes, a cardiovascular exercise must be aerobic, promoting the use of oxygen. We must sustain it for more than two minutes at a time without getting out of breath, like swimming or bicycling or running.

But, exercise and motion do not have to be fast, strenuous

or athletic to produce a variety of benefits. So don't let what you are doing, even if it is painting the garage, be "put down" as exercise. It can be a tonic for the mind and the body.

Another bonus for exercisers and body movers is a small loss in weight. A 200-pound person expends only 350 to 400 calories per hour doing active exercise, so it will take seven or eight hours of such exercise to lose one pound. The scale may show several pounds lost after just one or two hours of active exercise but this is water lost, not fat, and is soon restored. Any weight lost is a gain for longevity.

OTHER ERRORS OF OMISSION IN HEALTH CARE

Get plenty of good food, exercise, fresh air and sleep used to be the standard rule for longevity.

All four of these essentials are getting more and more difficult to come by. Refined food and the sedantary life are now accompanied by air pollution that limits the third necessity of long life and the late, late show. That limits the fourth.

Mankind is becoming more and more aware of air pollution and the need to limit the chemicals and gases poured into our atmosphere by factories and transportation. Perhaps the turnaround has come. But even so, it costs you years of life to live beside a heavily trafficked turnpike or in a smoke-filled neighborhood. Statistics show lung problems rise with proximity to this kind of air.

Even if I were to say, "Be aware of the air you breathe," many of you would not be able to do much about it. Pittsburgh is Pittsburgh. Toyko is Tokyo. But if something can be done, you need to do it.

Certainly, you can do something about your own air pollution. Use fewer chemical sprays as deodorants, insect repellants, dry cleaners, and hair preparations.

The New Hampshire Lung Association, with the help of federal funds, is enabling high school students to smoke in class in order to show them the harm that smoking inflicts on their bodies.

Classrooms are supplied with equipment that permits the

pupils to monitor heart rate, skin temperature, carbon monoxide in the bloodstream, and nervousness. Students are monitored before and after smoking and are able to witness their heart rate increase, carbon monoxide in the blood increase, skin temperature decrease, and nerve steadiness decrease.

By actually seeing the effects on their bodies in this way, smoking students are motivated to cut down or give it up. Nonsmokers stay that way.

The American Heart Association is taking up the cudgel against smoking again. New studies show that smoking is even more damaging to the heart than to the lungs. Of the estimated 325,000 Americans who die premature deaths because of cigarettes each year, over 100,000 of these are early deaths due to heart attacks.

Taking up smoking is a sin of commission. Not giving up the habit is a sin of omission. Have you committed either sin or both?

Reprogram yourself to be a nonsmoker. Here is how:

- Relax.
- Give yourself instructions to smoke your first cigarette later tomorrow and with longer intervals between cigarettes.
- Tell yourself you no longer need the smoke, that your lungs require fresh air.
- See yourself complying as you end your relaxation.

You can continue this tapering-off process until you are smoking at only a fraction of your previous rate. Then it will be easier to give yourself instructions that you need never smoke again.

SLEEPING YOUR WAY TO BETTER HEALTH

This subject of living longer involves the whole spectrum of health. I am tempted to talk about so many dos and don'ts that it can become totally disorganized and confusing.

Don't take appetite suppressants to lose weight. Most contain a drug fenfluramine found to kill brain cells in research animals. With dosages reduced to reflect the amounts used by humans, fenfluramine was found to increase pain from injury, produce insomnia and interfere with sexual hormone development.

Don't stay long on liquid protein. It is not only devoid of other nutrients necessary for the body to use the protein, as we mentioned before, but the protein is missing a few amino acids in many makes and is therefore zero protein.

Don't stay out in the sun too long. Noonday summer sun can cause skin cancer quite rapidly, compared to other times of the day or year. Skin cancers comprise more than half of all the new cases of malignancy diagnosed each year, but only about two percent of the cases of skin cancer are the dangerous malignant melanomas that are capable of spreading to other parts of the body. Use a sunscreen preparation not a suntan lotion if you must be in hot sun for an hour or more, less for sensitive skins.

Back to the late, late show.

It is not just nightlife and television that rob us of sleep. It is also stress.

There is no rule of thumb that dictates how much sleep we need. Most people accept eight hours as normal. But there are people who get along with five or four hours. Edison was said to sleep only four hours. He managed to acquire over 1,200 U. S. patents and lived to 84.

The major threat to health lies in lying awake. When you cannot fall asleep right away or wake up in the middle of the night and toss, you raid the refrigerator or you take a sleeping pill. There are millions of insomniacs in the United States and sleeping pills are a multi-million dollar business.

You won't find sleeping pills in areas of the world where actuarial tables crumble. Long-lived peoples are not usually pill poppers of any kind.

If you have trouble falling asleep, occasionally or habitually, ask yourself the question: "What is keeping me awake?" The answer will like be: "I am keeping me awake."

There are mental techniques to keep you from thinking about the things that are concerning you. One of the oldest is counting sheep. If you have ever lied awake counting imaginary sheep as they jumped over a split rail fence, you know how boring this can be. But that is the key. Mental techniques to hasten sleep must have enough methodology to keep you mentally occupied and be boring enough to send the conscious mind into the retreat we call sleep.

The relaxation techniques given you in the previous chapter help you to move nearer to sleep. When you get relaxed, count backward slowly from 100 to 1, seeing the numbers in your imagination, rather than whispering them or repeating them mentally. Most people who use this method never get below 80. The next thing they know it is morning.

MAINTAINING AWARENESS
OF POSSIBLE HEALTH THREATS

With the realization of the absence of roughage in our diet and the health problems it has been causing, many large bakeries have been marketing "high fiber" bread. People buy the bread thinking they are getting the roughage part of the grain that was previously removed. Now it has been disclosed that what one or more of the bakeries has been doing is using pulverized wood pulp. In one case this wood comprised one-third the weight.

The Canadian government has banned the use of bread manufactured with micro crystallene cellulose, the scientific name for what really amounts to sawdust. In the United States, although the Food and Drug Administration is studying the effects of eating wood pulp, no decision has been made to ban it as of this writing.

I hope your awareness of possible threats to your health has been increasing as you proceed along these pages. The ultimate responsibility for your good health does not lie with the food manufacturers and suppliers, nor with their ad agencies, nor with the government, nor with the health care profession. It lies with you.

In a recent poll some 60 percent replied that they prefer "natural" on food labels. We are becoming more aware.

Yet, Congressman Robert Walker of Pennsylvania recently worked a few days in a food store and found that food stamp recipients were squandering their stamps on junk food like candy, soft drinks, and cake. He called this an evasion of the spirit of the food stamp program which was to help supply nutritious food to the needy.

Congress has a chance to insulate our people from junk foods wherever government subsidy is provided. Recently, it took such action by passing legislation giving the Secretary of Agriculture the authority to approve all food sold in on school grounds in competition with the federal school lunch program.

As a result, there is a good chance that the traditional foods that go into lunchroom vending machines, like soft drinks, potato chips, and candy bars will be replaced with more nutritious foods like dried fruit, raisins, apples, granola bars, nuts and seeds.

Of course, the problem still rests with you and me. If children refuse to buy what is in the vending machine because it is not candy, the availability of nutrition will not be effective. Taste buds hypnotized by sugar need to be dehypnotized. This takes re-education and teaching by example.

The United States is going the fast-food way. The names Magoo, Col. Sanders and McDonald's are becoming bywords. It is estimated that Americans now eat one-third of their meals out and that by the end of the 1980's this will rise to one-half. Most of these away-from-home meals are at fast food drive-ins and outlets. Most of that food eaten is fried or on white bread. Much of the rest is sugary drinks, pies and cake.

Not a minimum daily Vitamin A requirement in a carload.

De-hypnotizing ourselves from junk foods, fast or slow, starts with awareness. It continues with recognizing the food clues that trigger eating unhealthy food. These clues are on television and on radio. They beckon to us from signs and billboards. They reach out to us from boxes and packages.

Counteract commercials with simple affirmations like "Garbage!" Put a big, red mental "X" across any sign for junkie munchies. Step on the gas not the brake when passing those roadside golden arches.

NEW AND UNEXPECTED HEALTH THREATS

Linus Pauling put his scientific neck on the block when he opposed nuclear testing. Each test risked 100,000 deformed babies, he claimed, and many more cases of cancer. He was nearly done in professionally. He was harrassed by government and blackballed by his own colleagues who feared their own harrassment. Today, what he once was claimed disloyal for believing is government policy.

It may have been unpopular for us to berate junk foods years ago, but today it is the accepted thing and producers are scrambling to make food more nutritious.

Our awareness must be ever alert. We must be vigilantes in the fight against health sappers.

Workers in the nuclear industry exposed routinely to small amounts of radiation thought to be safe are taking a second look. Now, after 13 years of small amounts of radiation, it appears those small amounts are adding up to a fatal disease—cancer.

Here again, those in the industry and holding government related jobs in that industry are jumpy about being involved in the results of the study. Jobs and contracts are in jeopardy. Nevertheless, the statistics point to a conclusion that humans are 20 times more vulnerable to radiation-induced cancer than has been believed.

You are not in that nuclear industry. But you are surrounded by new electronic and radiation devices. Be aware. Use caution.

Are micro-wave ovens safe? What do they do to the minerals and vitamins in food. Is the protein "cooked" in a micro-wave oven fully assimilable? Full studies have not been made. Safety standards may be in error. A little harm over the years, undetected, may go a long way toward being critical harm.

Ask these questions about every new environmental factor, be it a cooking appliance or utensil, or a new food, or new cosmetics, drugs and toilet preparations.

Ask these questions about new inventions, new home attachments and comforts.

Ask these questions about new medical approaches to specific problems.

A few drinks of liquor are not dangerous to your health, but four drinks within a two-hour period, if you weigh 100 pounds, increases your chances of having an accident if you drive by 700 percent.

Combinations of safe things can produce unsafe things. Liquor and driving. Coke and aspirin. Sedatives and liquor.

Recently, a Brandeis University psychologist made an accidental discovery that may someday be offered as a longevity device for humans. The psychologist, Jerome Wodinsky, wanted to study the behavior of the male octopus after his sex glands were removed. He decided to first try removing the sex glands of the female octopus because, after the egg laying process, the female dies anyway.

However, instead of dying, the female octopus without her sex glands began to eat and grow. It went on living and doubled its life span.

Some years from now, you may be offered that choice: to have your sex glands removed and add years to your life.

That's quite a price to pay for extra years. But it might be symbolic of the fact that we have to give up certain pleasures to live longer.

Chapter 13

How Your Mind
Can Add Years to Your Life

The mind can make us sick.

The mind can make us well.

The first of these statements has been known for nearly fifty years, but only in recent years has medical science appreciated the mind's vast implications even for bacterial and viral diseases.

The second of these two statements is just emerging to take its place in man's understanding and hopefully in his evolution.

Your mind must stop making you sick. You have learned how to handle stress and anxiety. You relax, close your eyes and give your mind instructions which insulate you from stress.

Your mind must now start making you even more healthy. You do it the same way. You relax, close your eyes and give your mind instructions which make you more youthful, more attractive, and more vibrant.

Miss Terrie M. was a sort of junior executive in a television studio. An alive, good looking young woman, she came to my office in abject despair over a broken affair.

"It is not my first," she admitted. "How do I get off this treadmill. It's ruining my health."

She had dark rings under her eyes and her hands shook as she lit a cigarette. I could see she was a likely candidate for other health problems. "Headaches?" I asked. "Upset stomachs?" She nodded twice.

I helped Terrie relax physically and mentally and to give her brain three instructions that would ease the pain of her remorse and adjust her old programming that was causing her to behave in ways which were bound to lead to more emotional downfalls and even more serious physical symptoms.

The first instruction was pain relieving:

"I am in control of my emotions."

The second instruction was confidence restoring:

"I am a capable and attractive woman."

The third instruction put her more in tune with her world:

"This is a universe in which order prevails,
and in which I take my harmonious place."

Terrie was instructed to relax and reinforce these instructions three times a day. She left the office obviously feeling no pain. Within three days of self-programming, she was sleeping better and the physical symptoms of her emotional stress were gone.

The second and third instructions took a bit longer to work. But she did not have another affair. Her next "affair" was a marriage.

HOW WE PROGRAM OURSELVES TO DIE

We are always relaxing and giving our brain instructions. Take a look at Jim over there. He is day-dreaming. If you had entry to his thoughts, he is figuring out how long he has to retire and whether his income will last until his death. He is going by the figures he remembers from the interest tables and the actuarial tables. He sees himself living to 75. He thinks he is stealing a few extra years.

What he is really doing is programming himself to die.

A professional golfer sees the tee. He addresses the ball. When he looks up, he sees only the flag 300 yards away. You and I see the flag, too, but we also look to the left and we see the water hazard and we look to the right and we see the rough. We program ourselves for error.

Not so the pro. That is why he is a pro.

We see the actuarial tables. We see people getting gray, wrinkled, and bent. We see people die in their sixties and seventies. We program ourselves for error.

Meanwhile in Hunza land, adults see people young looking, energetic and erect, living well over the century mark. They program themselves for longevity.

They are the pros in the game of life.

PLAYING THE GAME OF LIFE TO WIN

You can eat nothing but "wonder" foods with plenty of vitamins and minerals. You can get plenty of sleep, exercise, pure water and pure air and still die young if . . .

If you worry yourself to death.

Death itself is what many people worry about. They fear disease and lower their resistance with this very fear. They panic with every pain and sap their strength with panic. They get "up tight" with every minor malfunction and throw the organs out of balance with their tension.

There is a medical doctor in Texas who has been helping cancer patients in an unusual way. Dr. Carl Simonton started this at Travis Air Force Base some five years ago, as a radiologist. Statistics began to show cancer being cured at a faster and more successful rate at Travis than at other bases. What is this unusual way?

Dr. Simonton has his patients relax and imagine they are inside their bloodstream helping to get rid of the dead and dying cancer cells following a radiation treatment.

The mind can make us well, just as it can make us sick.

Picturing with the mind is a creative act. Persist with a picture and it brings about the very picture. Franklin D. Roosevelt realized that the depressed economy of the early nineteen thirties was at least partially due to depressed people. "We have nothing to fear but fear itself," he reminded Americans. And it is so.

People do not like to take the blame for their own problems, much less their own health. Most of the cancer patients who flocked to Texas to investigate the Simonton method never stayed when they found out it relied largely on their own relaxation and visualization.

You need to back up the Longevity Diet with a consciousness of longevity.

To have a consciousness of longevity, you need to believe in the "wonder" foods and you need to believe in the importance of your own thoughts.

That is how you can play the game of life to win.

You can use your thoughts to win additional years.

You can use your thoughts to win additional wealth.

You can use your thoughts to win additional success in any field.

THE ADVANTAGES OF POSITIVE IMAGERY

I am a clinical hypnologist. I help people to relax and accept new mental pictures to replace the old. And I see their lives conform to these new pictures.

It can be a picture of themselves as a non-smoker. They then become a non-smoker.

It can be a picture of themselves with a better complexion. Their skin improves.

It can be a picture of themselves more successful in their job. They become more effective and more successful.

But more important for survival, it can be a picture of themselves in better health.

These positive mental pictures at a deeply relaxed level—which is basically what hypnotism and self-hypnotism entails—helps with many health problems.

Surgeons can operate without giving the patient anesthesia. Childbirth is made easier. Tooth extraction is painless. Gastrointestinal and respiratory ailments disappear. There are actually no bounds. I have been called into an operating room by a surgeon when a patient is hemorrhaging and even though that patient was under a general anesthesia, I have been able to "command" the hemorrhaging to stop. And it did. It did because, even under anesthesia, the brain is aware and obeys.

The hypochondriac who imagines he is sick is helping the body to get that way and can eventually prove to everybody he was right. Every time you visualize yourself getting sick, you are creating that illness.

The mind that fears all kinds of illness is digging a very real grave.

You cannot win the game of life that way.

The way to win it is to abandon all fear and put health-building confidence in its place.

The body's natural state is: perfect.

We interfere.

The power of thinking positively does its best work by ending the negative thinking. This permits the body to perfect itself.

This is so important to you that I would be remiss if I did not give you ways to change your negative thoughts.

Call it self-hypnosis if you will. There are now so many new programs that bring about mind-body cooperation through relaxation and visualization that the old names for this practice get blurred.

It is a fact though that society has opened up in recent years to now accept hypnosis and self-hypnosis, the grand-daddy of all self-help techniques.

Hypnosis and self-hypnosis are accepted today as an extension of the so-called human potential movement.

You call it what you will. Just . . .

Relax the body and mind. Then see yourself as you want to be.

It is very much like daydreaming.

HOW TO RELAX AND PERPETUATE GOOD HEALTH

I have already given you relaxation techniques for combatting stress. You can relax any way that seems comfortable for you to do so, but since deep relaxation brings about results faster, you may want to add to your repertoire of relaxation techniques.

Here are a few. They are in the preferred order of use. Try them. Select those that are right for you:

- Stare at a point on the ceiling or wall turning your eyes up but not your head. Try to keep from blinking. When your eyes feel like closing, in a few seconds, permit them to close.

- With your eyes closed, take a few deep breaths.
- Be aware of your breathing in normal rhythm for a minute or so.
- Check out your body from head to toe to make sure every part is relaxed. Start by relaxing your scalp, then go to your forehand, cheeks, jaw, neck, shoulders, etc. all the way to your ankles and toes.
- Count backwards from ten to one or from 25 to one.
- Imagine you are surrounded by a gray cloud through which no outside thoughts can penetrate.
- Imagine that you are in a peaceful garden or other place that you find relaxing.
- Imagine you are facing a blackboard on which the numbers one to ten are written. As your mind wanders to an outside thought, get up mentally and erase a number, knowing that when all the numbers are erased, your mind will be at rest.

The first five of these are ways to relax the body. The next three are ways to relax the mind.

Now that you are relaxed in body and mind, what do you do with your thoughts to perpetuate good health.

You "command," "instruct," or "suggest" that you be the way you want to be. You say it with words. You back up the words with mental pictures.

Here are a few general statements and pictures you can use:

- "I accept good health as a natural state for me. It is right. I see myself in topnotch health." (See it.)
- "I am calm and relaxed. I am free of fear and worry. I do not get easily excited. I am serene and confident. This permits unlimited health and energy to manifest in me." (See it.)
- "I am in perfect health. My organs function flawlessly. Every system of my body is in balance." (See it.)

Now here are some specific statements to counteract unwanted symptoms or conditions:

- For a cold or respiratory ailment—"My resistance is high. I am not affected by other people's colds or warnings. I am resourceful, capable, and strong." (See yourself breathing freely and healthfully.)

- For skin rashes, blemishes, or allergies: "These blemishes will disappear (or warts will fall off, or erupting will recede and heal, etc.). I do not have them. I am ridding myself of them. My skin is getting better and better. I see my skin clear and attractive." (See it so.)
- For headache: "I have no need of a headache. I am calm and relaxed. When I end my relaxation, the discomfort in my head will be greatly relieved. (Repeat in a few minutes until gone.)
- For stomach upset: 'I can identify the emotional problem that affects my stomach. Now my stomach can be restored to healthy state. It is getting better and better, operating normally, free of pain or discomfort. I see it perfect. I feel fine." (See it.)

Always end your relaxation session "seeing" yourself perfect. Reinforce by repetition, three times a day at least. As the symptoms fade, reinforce with a general instruction, not a specific instruction for that symptom. You can select from the three given above or this:

"Every day in every way my health gets better and better. I reject negative attitudes and emotions. They do not affect me. I see myself in perfect health, radiating youth, vigor and vitality." (See it!)

HOW THE MIND CAN STALL OFF SENILITY

Most people equate aging with senility. The old persons' mind no longer is able to function normally. Old people are forgetful. Their minds wander. They are often incoherent.

However, older people do not have to get senile, and if they do, it can be reversed in half the cases.

Dr. Carl Eisdorfer, a University of Washington psychiatrist, reported to a recent seminar on Psycho Pathology that it is not true that old people suffer a permanent loss of mental faculties, that they become feeble-minded. He said what we call senility is often a cognitive deficiency, meaning that they have not been exercising their minds enough.

Such people need to be kept alert and involved. A number of programs are being conducted now to provide interest for Senior Citizens. Dr. Eisdorfer recommends television programs like Sesame Street revised for older people. He recommends that they keep learning. Even playing pinball machines is cognitive exercise, he says.

We need to keep the mind active before senility can occur. "To rest is to rust" applies just as much to the mental as to the physical, and maybe more.

People need to be active and creative. Those who are freed to retire should find a second career or become more active in volunteer work. Turn your hobby into a business. Or travel, if you can. Join clubs and organizations and take an active role in them. Men and women who have professional or business skills might volunteer with their local Service Corps of Retired Executives (SCORE), a volunteer arm of the U. S. Small Business Administration, for counseling people in small business.

There is a trauma to retirement. It says, "That is it, brother. All that's left for you to do now is get ready to die."

Not so. First, do not retire if you can help it. Second, if you are forced to retire, gear up for new experiences as if you were just coming out of college.

THE BRAIN'S RULE IN AGING

If you were to look at the brain under a powerful microscope, you would see a network of neurons or information centers, each one sending out many tiny fingers to contact neighboring neurons.

It was formerly believed that this network was totally complete prior to birth. But now scientists have found that the real brain growth spurt comes in the first few years of a child's development.

This brain growth can be hindered by poor nutrition and a lack of challenge or experiences.

Right at this moment, inadequate nutrition is causing lasting brain damage to children in those parts of Africa and South America where famine and poverty prevail. You can see how the cycle feeds itself: Periods of poor nutrition starve young children's brains. They never develop to full mental capacity and seem relegated to more poverty.

Good nutrition is always important, from prenatal months to old age. But it is critically important for age one and age two. Deprivation then is lasting. Watch those prepared baby foods. With today's blenders, you might want to think about preparing your baby's nutritional means yourself.

An impoverished social life is also damaging to the brain neurons of young children.

In one study using the Caldwell Inventory of Home Stimulation, it was found that children with a low frequency of adult contacts, voices heard, toys and games played with, and new activities were below their more active peers in mental and physical functioning.

The mind needs to be nourished as well as the body.

In 1976 there was a unique gathering in South Carolina. A meeting of that state's centenarians was held in Columbia under the auspices of South Carolina's Commission on Aging. Attending were 31 people aged 100 or more, with the oldest 108. Not able to attend were 130 other centenarians in the state. Centenarian Mrs. Josephine Matthews was given the state's outstanding older citizen award. A midwife who helped with the delivery of over 1,300 babies, she is still active in church and civic affairs.

This kind of activity could well be the golden key to golden years.

Cranial calisthenics like physical calisthenics are similar to empty calories. They are exercises in futility—full of the expenditure of energy but going nowhere.

The real benefit to the exercising of mind and body comes with the reaching for and attainment of meaningful results.

I vote against exercise for exercising sake—mental and physical. I vote for activity with a creative purpose—mental and physical.

For longevity's sake.

HOW TO KEEP ABREAST
OF LATEST SCIENTIFIC DEVELOPING ON AGING

Until recently, investigations into aging, both its mental and physical aspects, produced no clear-cut results. A multitude of fragments did not fit together into any big picture.

Today, that picture is beginning to emerge. However, it is not one picture but two.

First, there is the picture that focused scientific research is beginning to come up with.

Second, there is the picture that is emerging from the empirical data supplied by life itself.

The Longevity Diet and other longevity steps in this book are basically the latter, because it is life itself that teaches what is good for us and what is not.

It is not likely that this picture will change very much over the decades.

But it is likely that the first picture will not only come into better focus in the years ahead but may supply information that will provide even more bonus years than the Longevity Diet.

Scientific research in recent years has found, for instance, that the body's organs do not deteriorate dramatically with age. That conclusion had previously been made because researchers were looking at old humans and old animals that had died from disease.

The healthy heart does not age, nor does the healthy liver. One pumps blood just as well as it did nearly a century ago, the other disposes of alcohol and performs its many other functions just as well, too.

People like a Winston Churchill who continued to function in active positions long after they were supposed to have turned senile have endocrine systems and immune systems that have not been thrown out of balance by physical or mental excesses.

When you consider that our life expectancy averaged 47 years in 1900, you can appreciate how far we have come in extending life and how far we still may go in the years ahead within our life span. You need to keep abreast of these developments by reading magazines and newspapers and then writing to the agencies making the report for further information.

We are probably going to see more drugs come first. Our orientation right now is to medicine and surgery. It was not always like this and it may not always be so in the future. But meanwhile, science will be attempting to get a foothold on longevity in places where it is already familiar.

Science now knows that the principal aging centers are the

pituitary and hypothalamus glands. With aging comes a decline in the key brain chemical dopamine which acts as a nerve transmitter. This appears to affect the signals from the hypothalamus that controls the pituitary gland and its release of hormones.

The pituitary in turn triggers the release of thyroid hormones which play a key role in the development of the brain and in the cells of the immune system.

So it is a snowballing effect—we call it the aging cycle.

Will scientists learn how to stimulate these glands or synthesize its secretions? If so, stay on the Longevity Diet, but keep aware of this kind of progress.

It will be a while. But so far, working on these principles and others, scientists have doubled the life span of some animals.

By lowering the water temperature, tropical fish have been kept alive double their usual age. A reduced diet was part of this program.

Mice have had their lives prolonged with the chemical L-dopa, counteracting in part the brain's loss of dopamine. Incidentally, the "wonder" food wheat germ is one source of L-dopa.

An old mouse has also been rejuvenated by being surgically joined to a young mouse for a period, allowing the immune system of the old mouse to be "recharged."

Perhaps no physical stepping stone of aging stands out as starkly as the female menopause or "change of life." This occurs when the output of one female hormone estrogen is sharply curtailed and the output of another, prolactin, is increased. Again working with rats, scientists have restarted the estrogen production both with L-dopa and with the electrical stimulation of the hypothalamic areas of the brain.

These kinds of research have great promise for tomorrow. They bring you nothing today, except anticipation of that promise and activities that bear watching.

CURRENT YOUTHING TECHNIQUES
THAT HOLD PROMISE

When Dr. Maxwell Maltz, cosmetic surgeon, performed plastic surgery on prison inmates, correcting cauliflower ears, flattened noses, and other features typical of a convict look, these men when released had a lower rate of return to prison. Their self-image of being a convict was changed and so they changed.

There have been unnumerable instances of the same unexpected effect arising from face lifting and other costmetic surgery, such as skin abrasion, that leads to wrinkle and sag removal and a younger look.

A person who is made to look younger is being programmed to feel younger every time he looks in the mirror and by the reactions of other people.

Cosmetic surgery produces a synthetic beauty that is, therefore, more than skin deep. It can affect the psyche and the mind. And because the mind controls the body, youthful physical effects well outside the scope of the surgery can be triggered.

There are other youthing techniques that go deeper. Of course, there are the health spas all over the world. Some concentrate on weight, some on heart, some are "good" for whatever ails you."

But there are other techniques available. Some come and go. Many remain secret. One that has received widespread publicity recently has been a process known as chelation.

Chelation is a blood treatment purported to relieve poor circulation caused by hardening of the arteries. Improved circulation means more food to the body's cells. One place where it is given is Meadowbrook Hospital in Belle Chasse, Louisiana. Here, medical doctors perform a type of intravenous feeding using a compound called EDTA. It combines with inorganic calcium in the arteries but not with organic calcium.

Inorganic calcium clogs the arteries. Organic calcium moves to the teeth and bones, whenever needed.

The inorganic calcium combined with EDTA is then flushed out the kidneys. People who have been "chelated" have checked their urine and confirmed this calcium elimination. Circulation improves.

Although this treatment has been around for over twenty years, it is still considered relatively new. Chelation (pronounced "keylation") is not becoming standard practice by any means. Several hundred doctors have been trained to administer the treatment, but it is preventive medicine and therefore does not produce "cures" that make for dramatic medical practice results.

One positive step forward in even the minor acceptance of this treatment is in the recognition of a difference between organic and inorganic minerals. For decades natural health authorities have been proclaiming this difference but have been shouted down by scientists who say iron is iron and calcium is calcium.

The recognition of the importance of organic in mineral nutrition will end many, false nutritional claims, such as the claim that dry cereal has been iron fortified when iron filings have been dropped in the box. It will benefit us all as "organic" is accepted. It is the only nutritional language our body understands.

YOU CAN STAY ON THE PATH TO
THE FOUNTAIN OF YOUTH

Utah and Nevada are neighboring states. They share a similar climate, about the same degree of urbanization, altitude or topography, and about the same economic level.

Yet, the life expectancy in Utah is nearly four years longer than in Nevada—72.9 compared to 69. Medical economist Victor R. Fuchs made a study and found a startling excess of deaths in Nevada due to lung cancer and cirrhosis of the liver, the two major pitfalls of smoking and drinking.

Nevada is the gambling "capital" of the United States. With gambling come drinking and smoke-filled casinos.

Utah, on the other hand, is the Morman "capital" of the United States. Mormons are forbidden by their church to smoke or drink alcohol. Even tea, coffee, and soda with caffeine (like the "Coke" family) are not permitted.

You do not have to go to Nevada to suffer fatal lung or liver damage, any more than you have to become a Utah Mormon to live longer. The choice is yours wherever you are.

You can stay on the path to the Fountain of Youth by using the Longevity Diet as your compass and by applying common sense (gut feeling) rules to your steps.

It is your choice all the way. You can choose to live a Utah or Nevada type of life.

That's the long and the short of it.

FIFTEEN CHOICES
YOU CAN MAKE NOW FOR LONGER LIFE

The late W. C. Fields is still regarded as one of America's all-time great comedians. He was a heavy drinker. His drinking interfered with film production schedules and raised production costs. Fields purportedly deducted the cost of his two bottles of liquor a day as a business expense because, "I make my living as a comedian and I cannot be funny unless I drink."

Fields died at the height of his career. But his assassin—liquor—was his choice.

In a way, people who die of lung cancer also do so by choice. It is no big thing.

It is whether to light up or not. (One more won't make any difference.)

It is whether to use butter or margarine. (Butter tastes better.)

It is whether to eat pork or veal, cake or fruit.

It is a lot of little choices every hour of every day.

I would like you to make these choices in advance—now. Below are fifteen choices. The left column is the path to shortevity. The right column is the path to longevity.

If you choose all left-hand options, please leave this book to somebody in your will. Half left and half right-hand choices will probably leave you squarely on the actuarial tables. More right hand than left-hand choices will give you a chance for more years. All right-hand choices will very likely entitle you eventually to membership in a centenarian's club.

Shortevity	Longevity
I am a smoker.	I do not smoke.
I drink liquor frequently.	I drink moderately if at all.
Sweets, fats and starches are my favorite food.	Protein is my favorite food.
I pass up salad.	I eat salad everyday.
I eat anything I like.	I favor "wonder" foods.

I live to eat.	I count calories, eat to live.
Fruits? Vegetables? No thanks.	I say yes to fruits and vegetables.
I can't be bothered with vitamins.	I take vitamin C and B-complex daily.
Mineral supplements? No interest.	I take a general mineral supplement daily.
Pass the sugar.	Sugar? No thanks.
Pass the salt.	No salt, thanks.
Who needs sleep.	I sleep 7 or 8 hours a night.
Save your energy—ride.	Save your life—walk.
I'd rather be fat and jolly.	I'd rather be slender and alive.
Water rusts your pipes.	Pure water is the best thirst quencher.

When you have made your choices, you can help yourself live up to them by relaxing and mentally seeing yourself on that path.

See yourself a non-smoker, eating right, and living naturally. See a perpetual calendar in the picture with you.

See the pages turning—1980, 1990, 2000, 2010 . . . with you still young, vigorous, attractive and effective.

2020 . . . 2030 . . . 2040 . . .

Index